The 7 ESSENTIAL HAIRCUTS *for* WOMEN

COLORING BOOK

By NIKKI MORGAN ALLEN

Illustrated by MELANIE LA MAY and NIKKI MORGAN ALLEN

The 7 Essential Haircuts for Women - COLORING BOOK

Copyright © 2022 by Denise C Allen

All rights reserved.

Illustrated by Melanie La May and Nikki Morgan Allen
Book Cover and Formatting by Trisha Fuentes

No part of this book may be reproduced in any form or by any electronic or mechanical means, including information storage and retrieval systems, without written permission from the author, except for the use of brief quotations in a book review.

ISBN: 979-8-9850397-3-3 Paperback

This coloring book is dedicated to the people who put the color in my life...

Bob Allen
Joey Louis
Morgan Louis
James Allen
Diane Morgan
Ray Morgan
Trella Bowling

Thank you all!!!

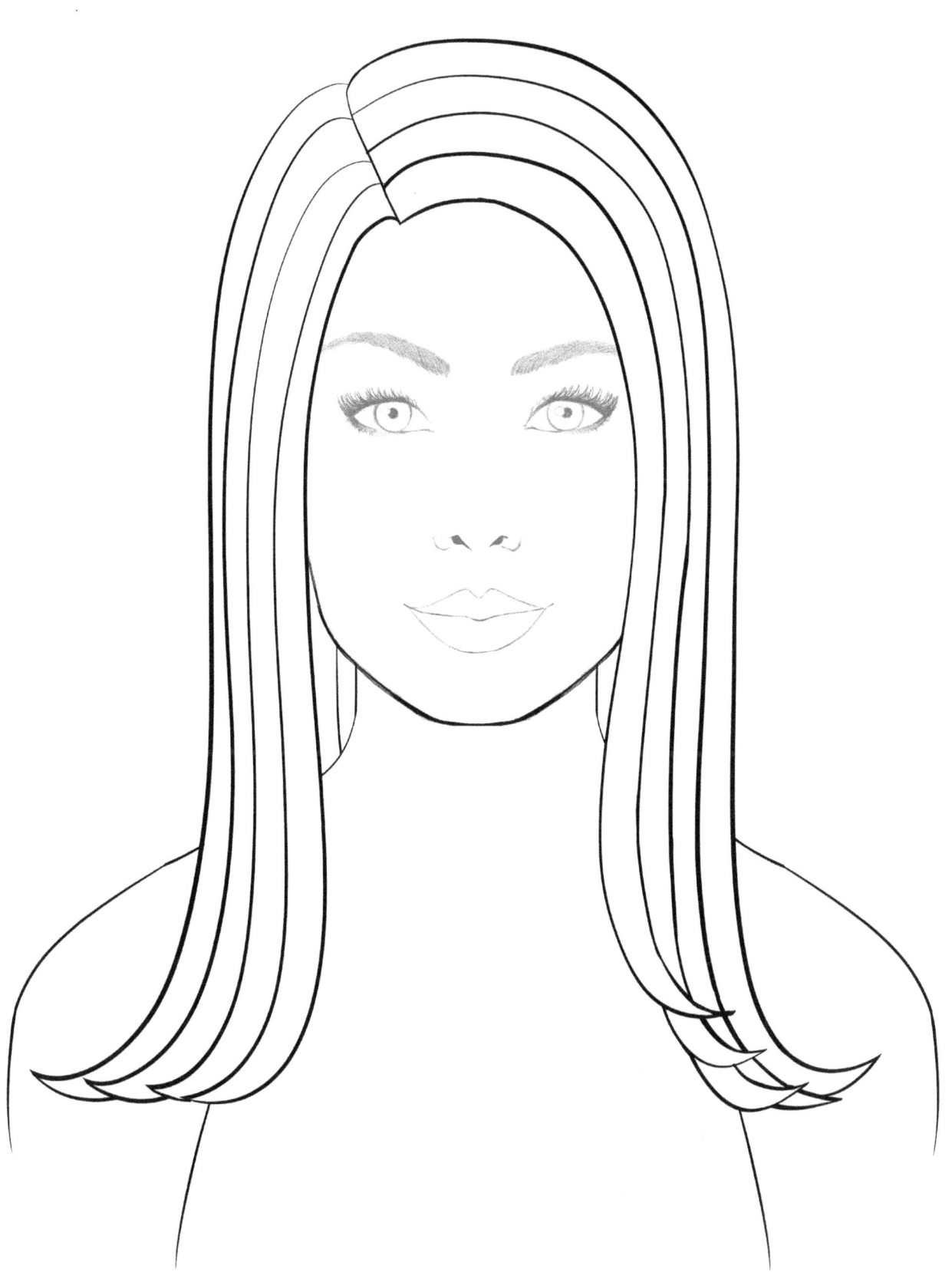

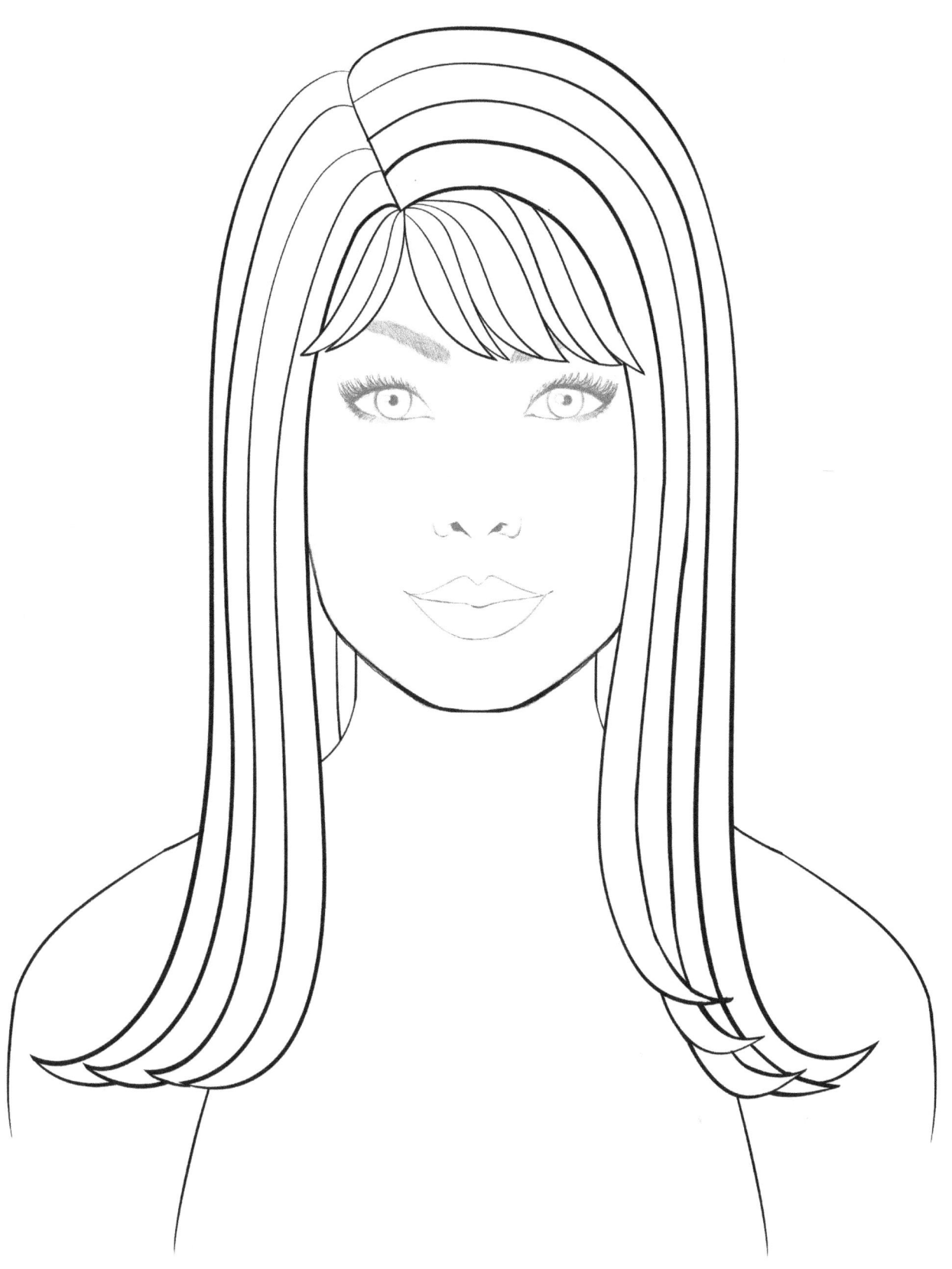

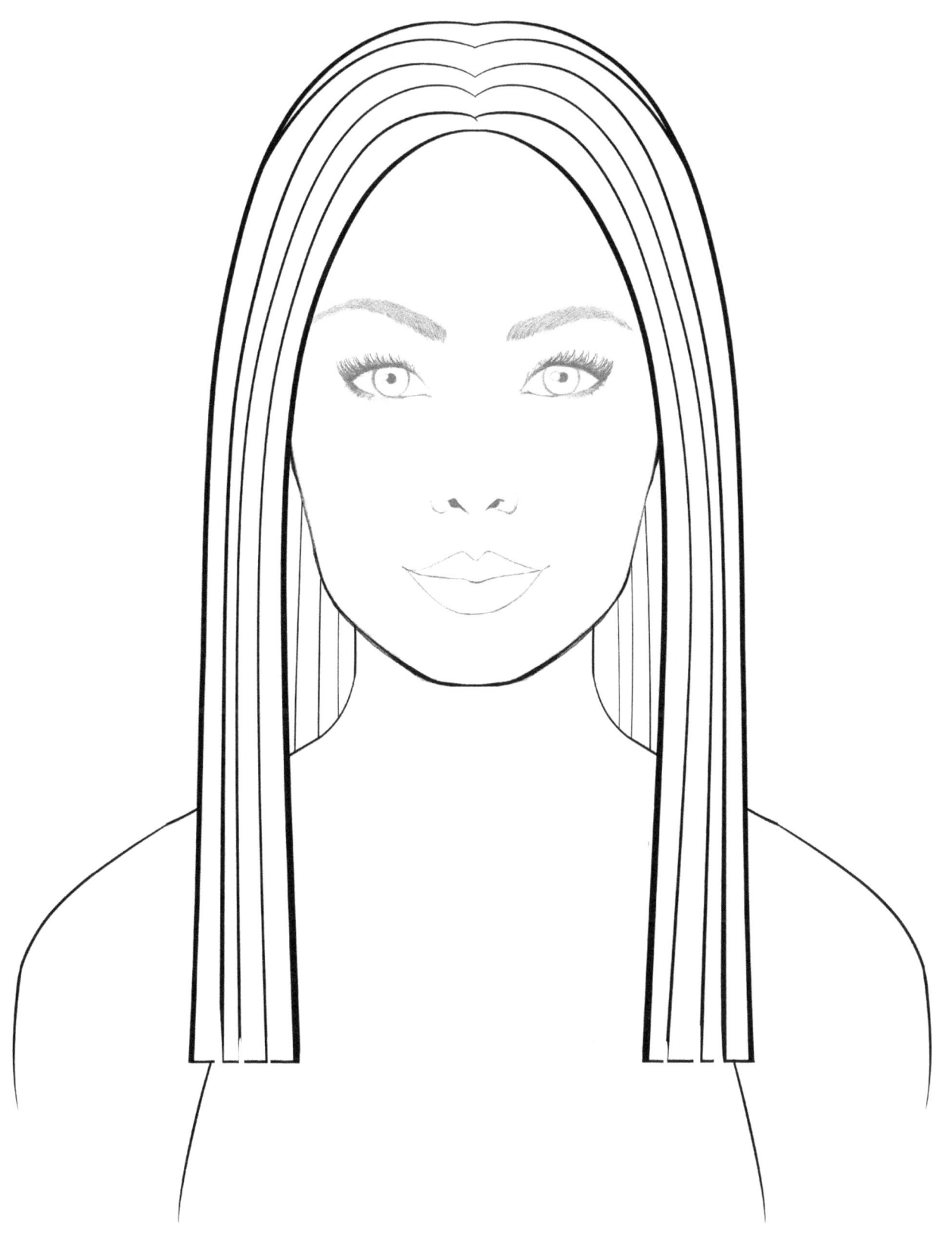

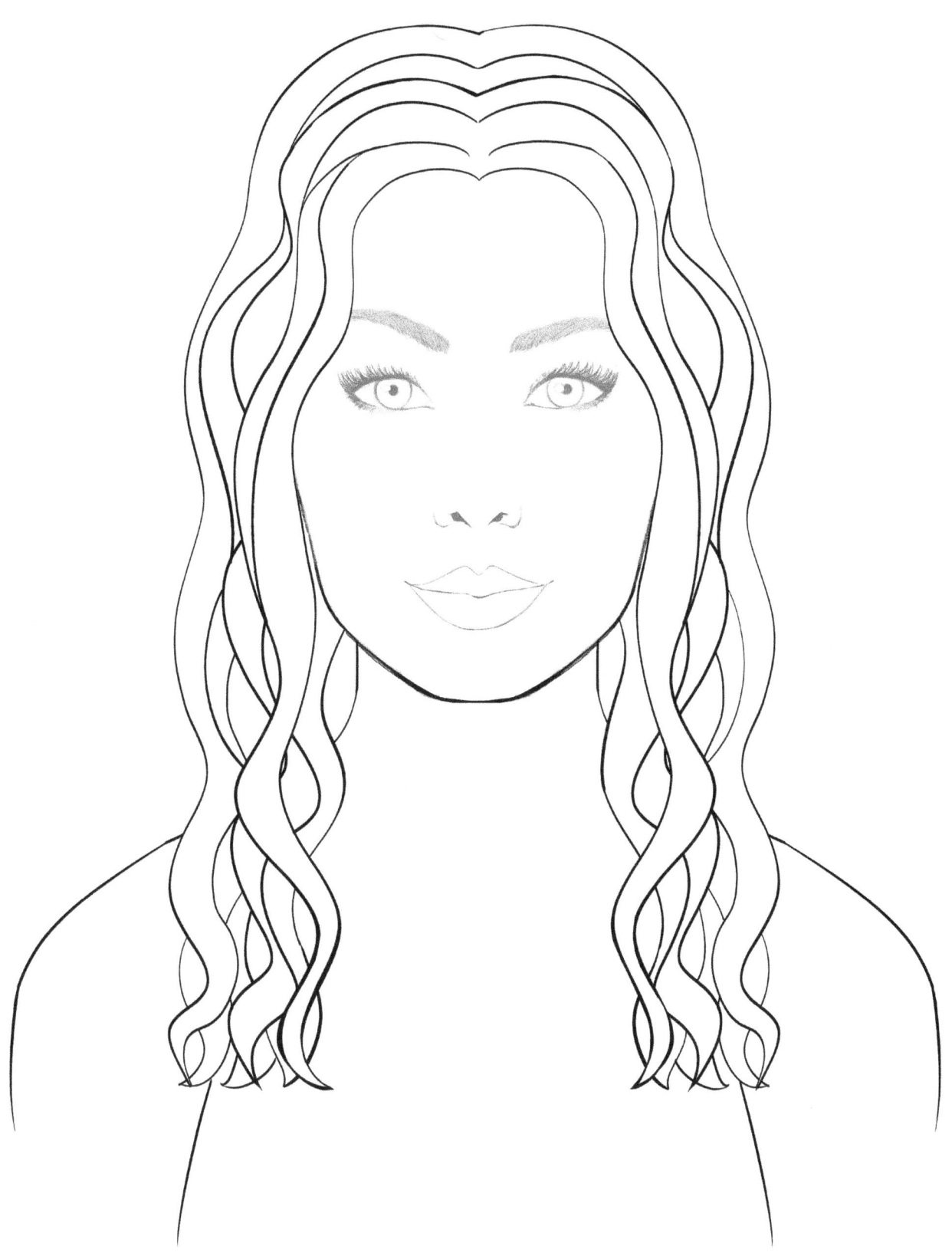

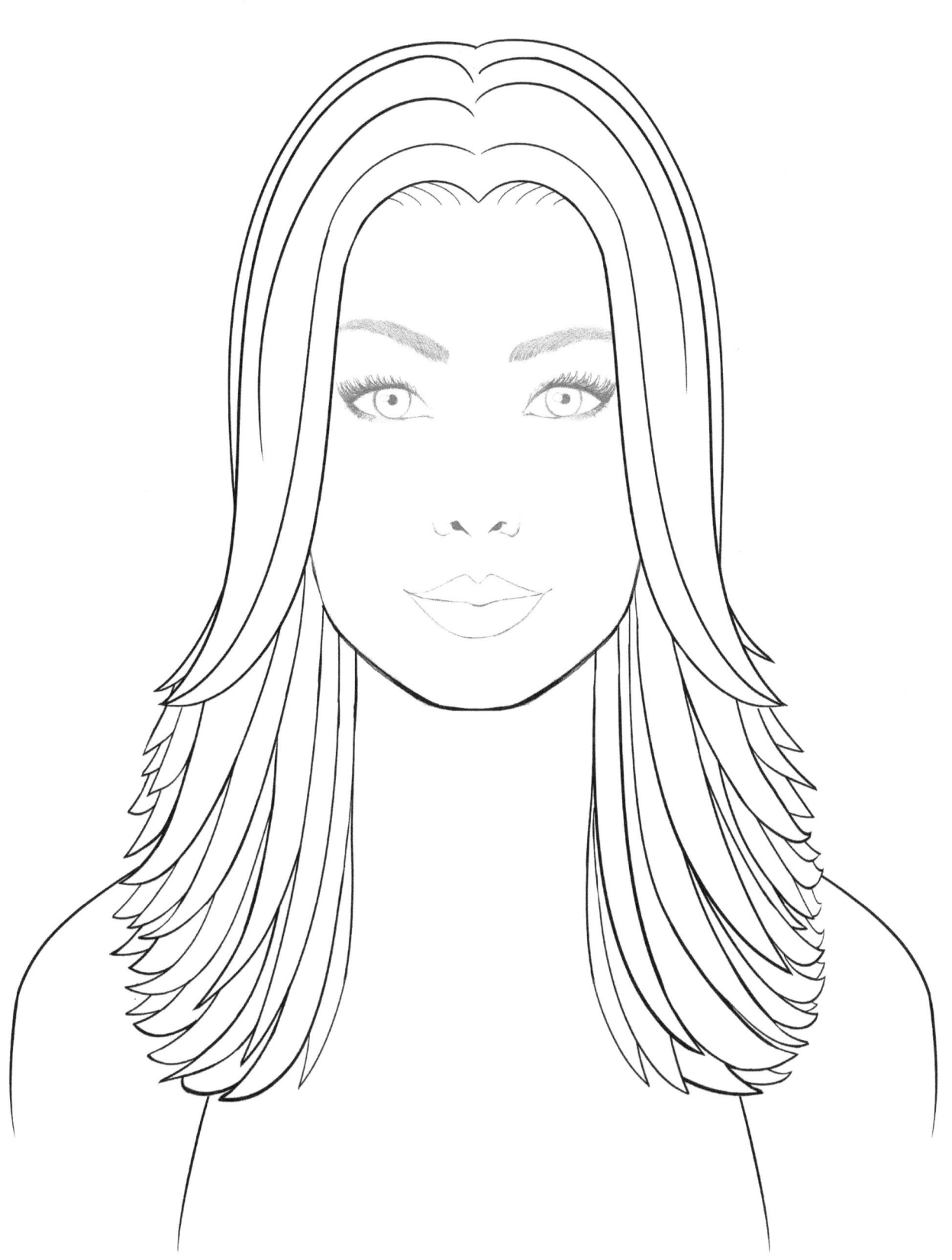

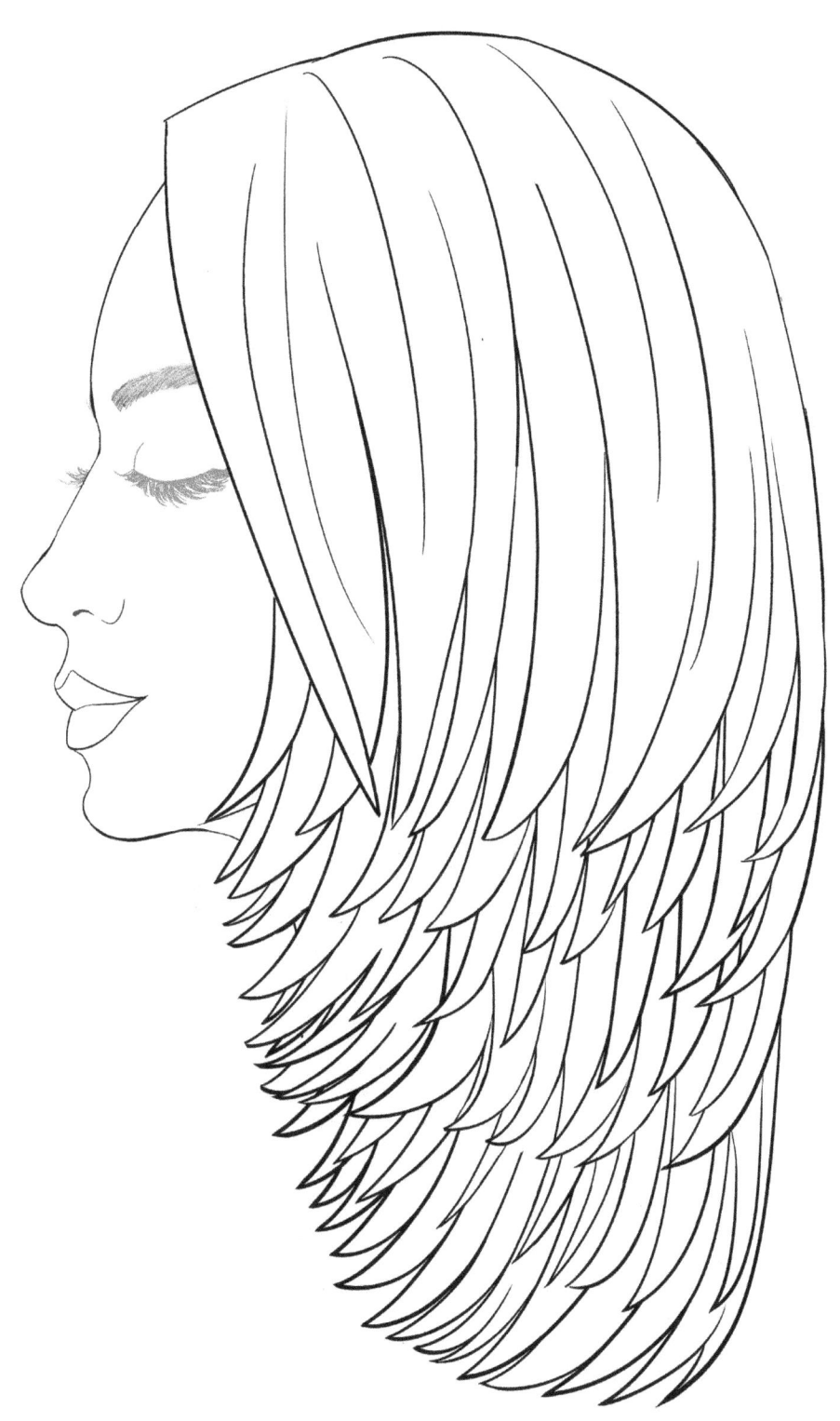

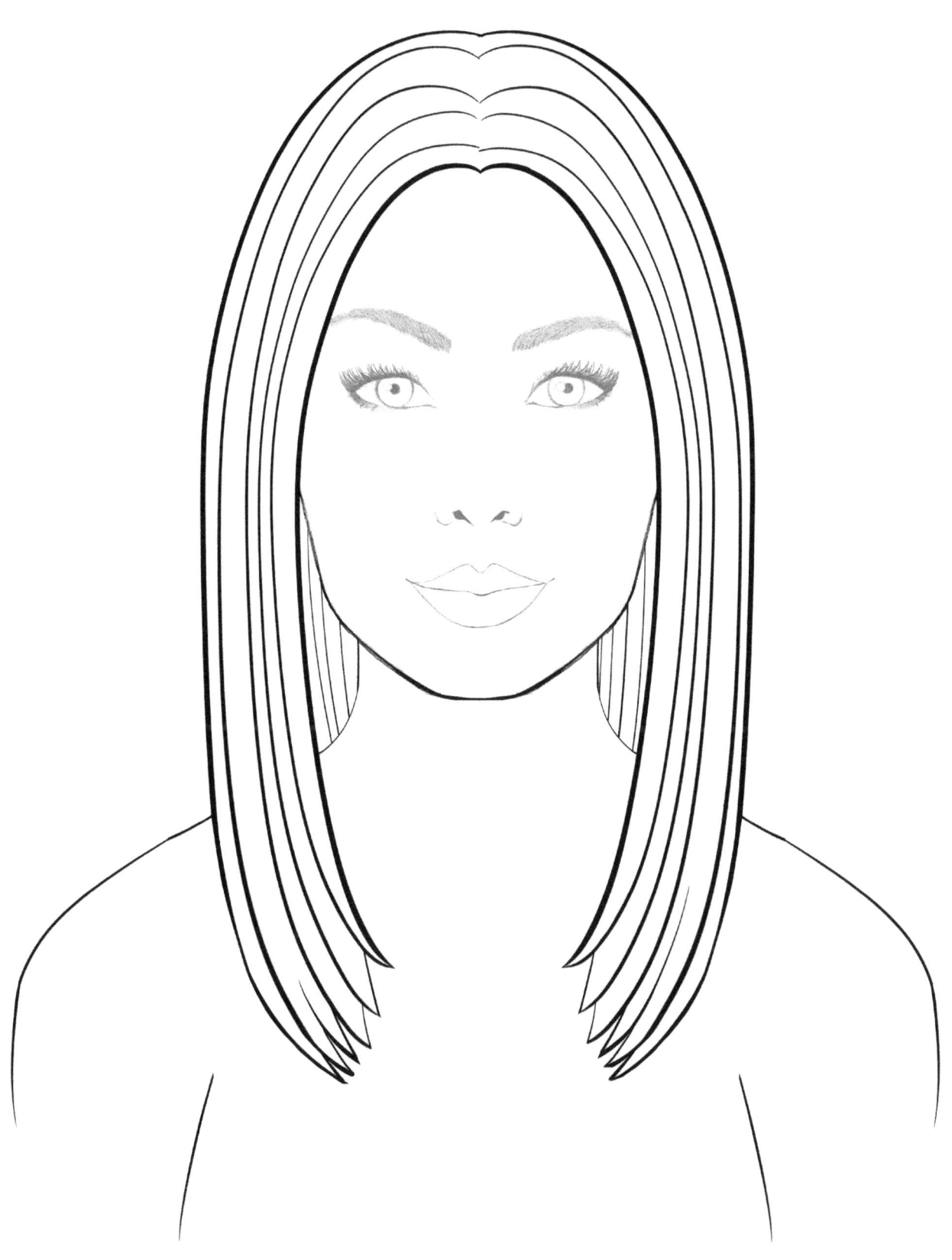

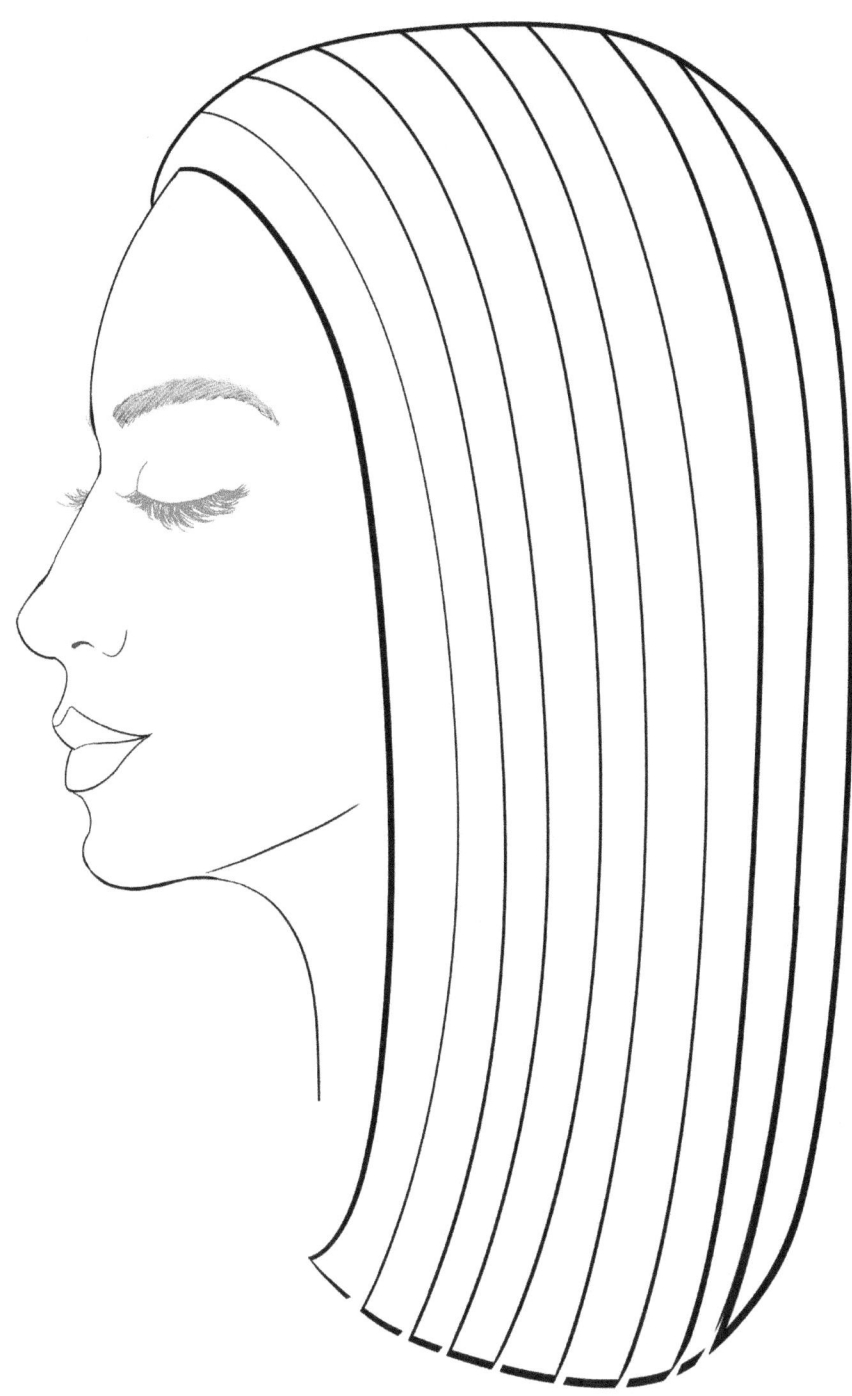

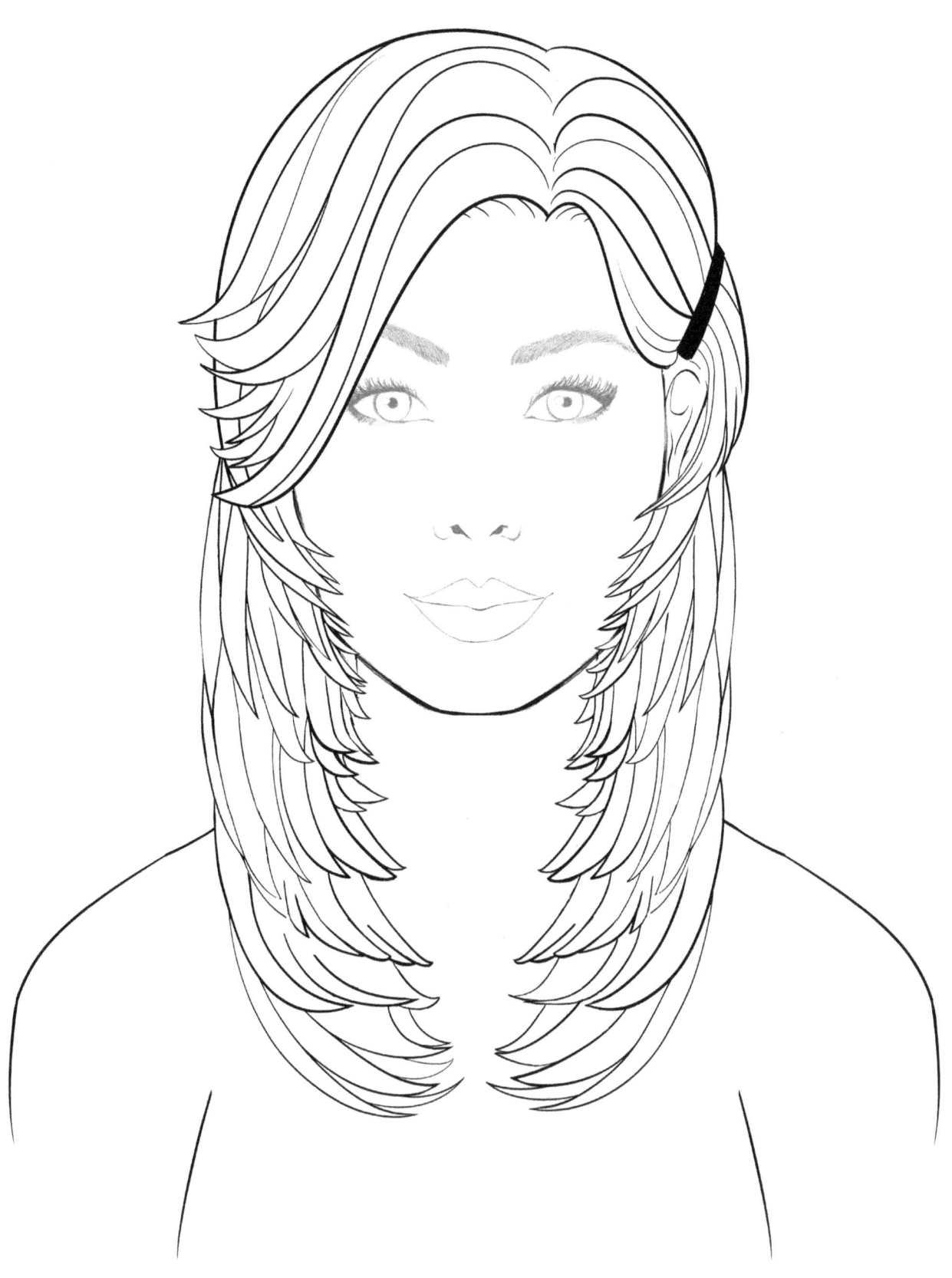

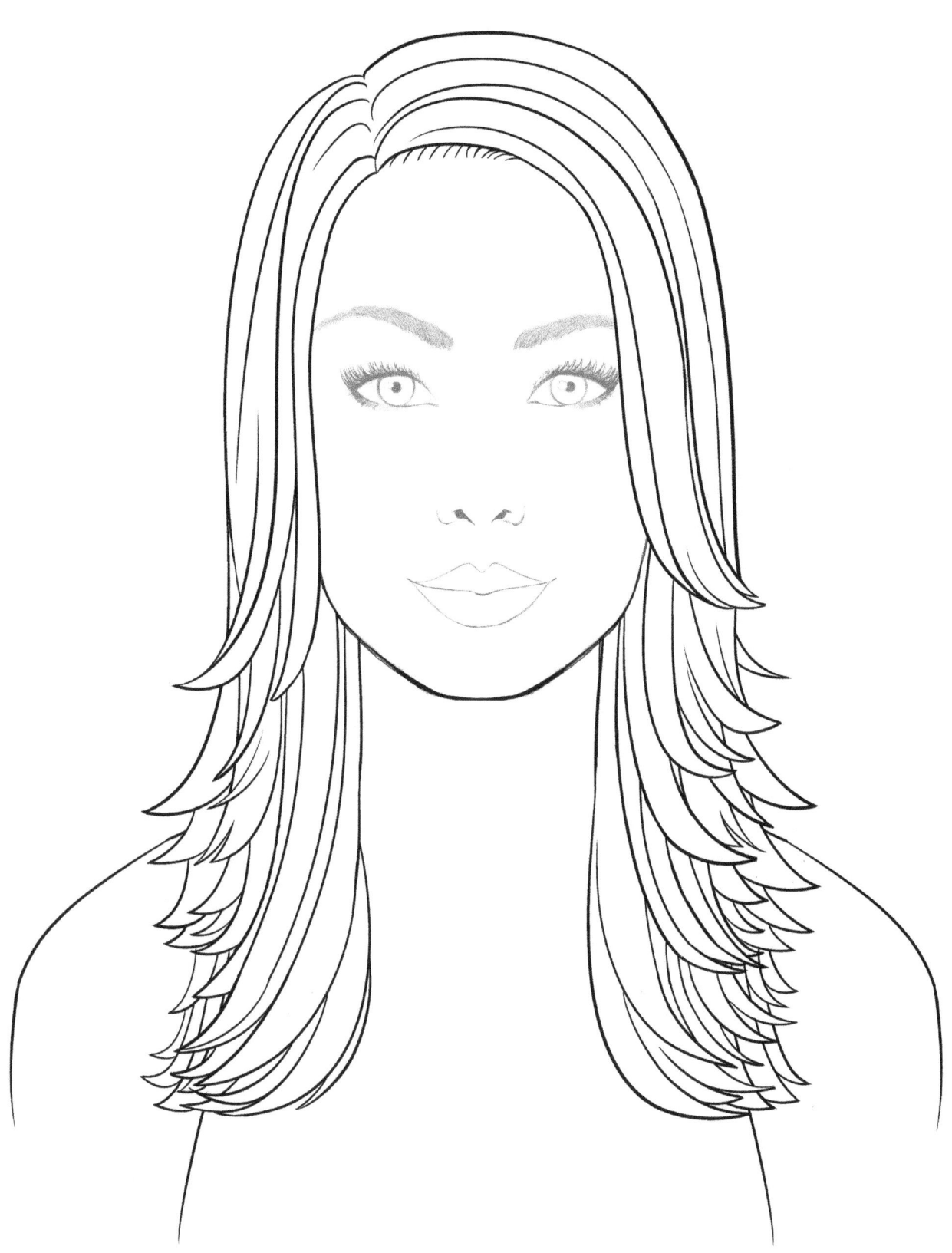

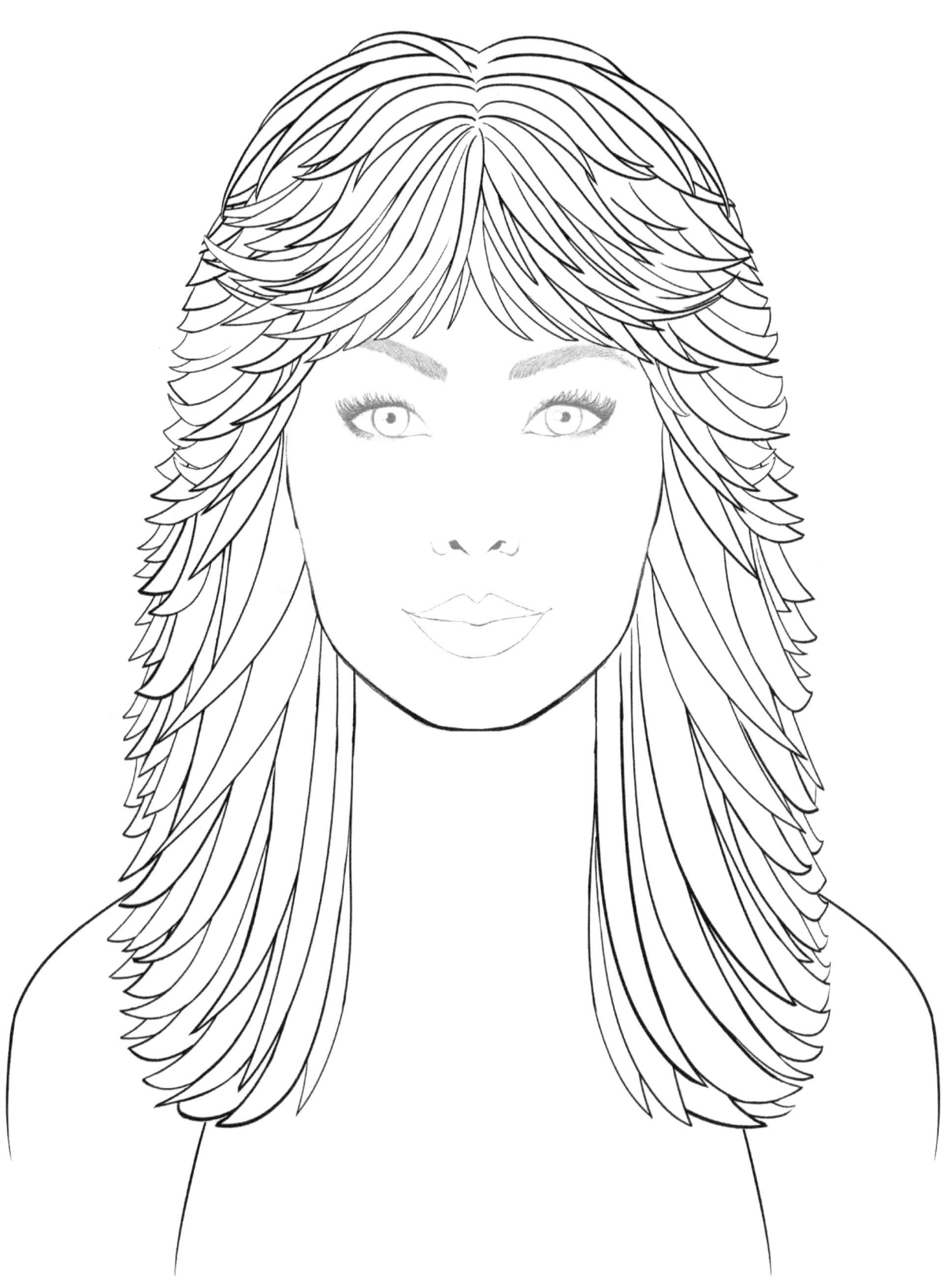

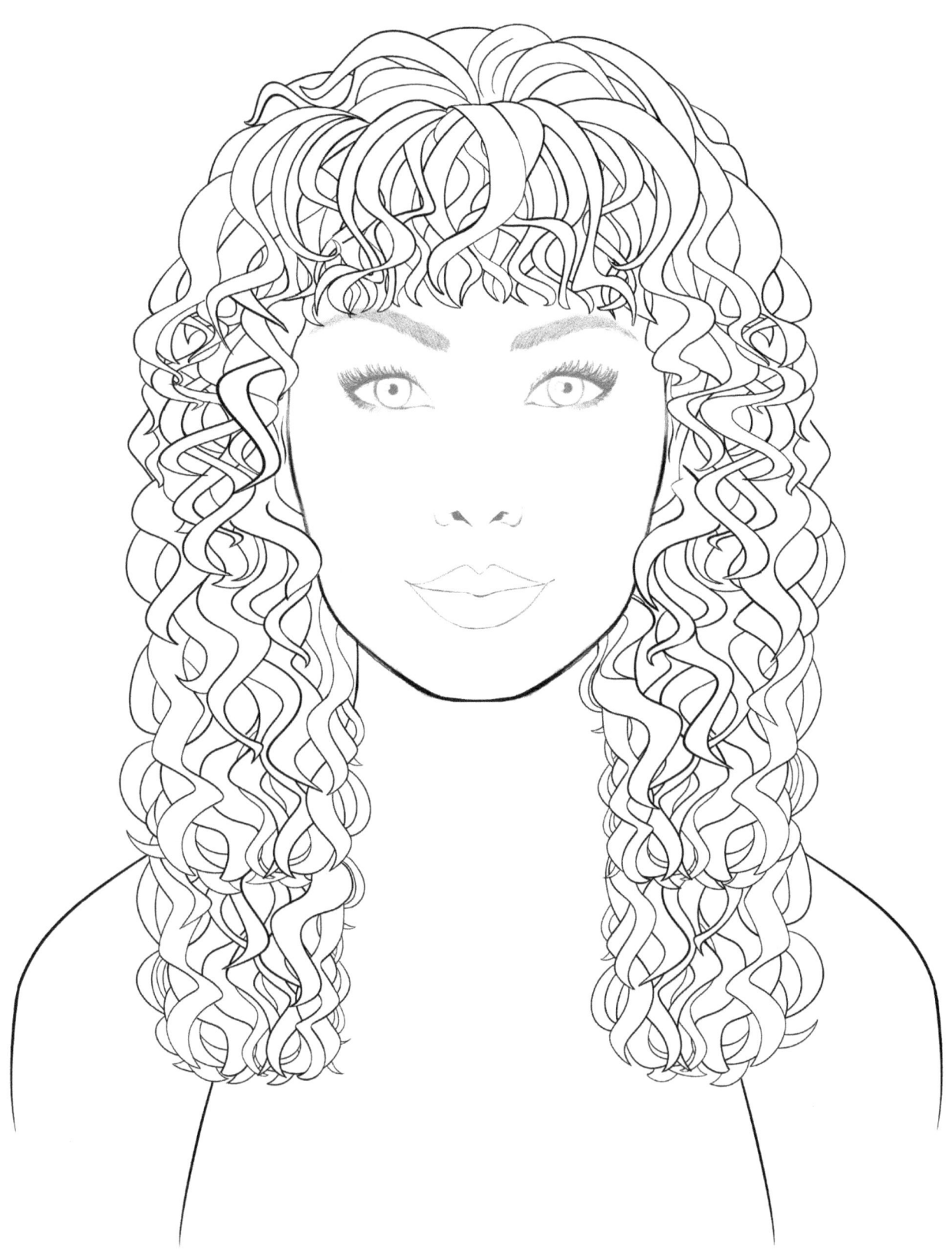

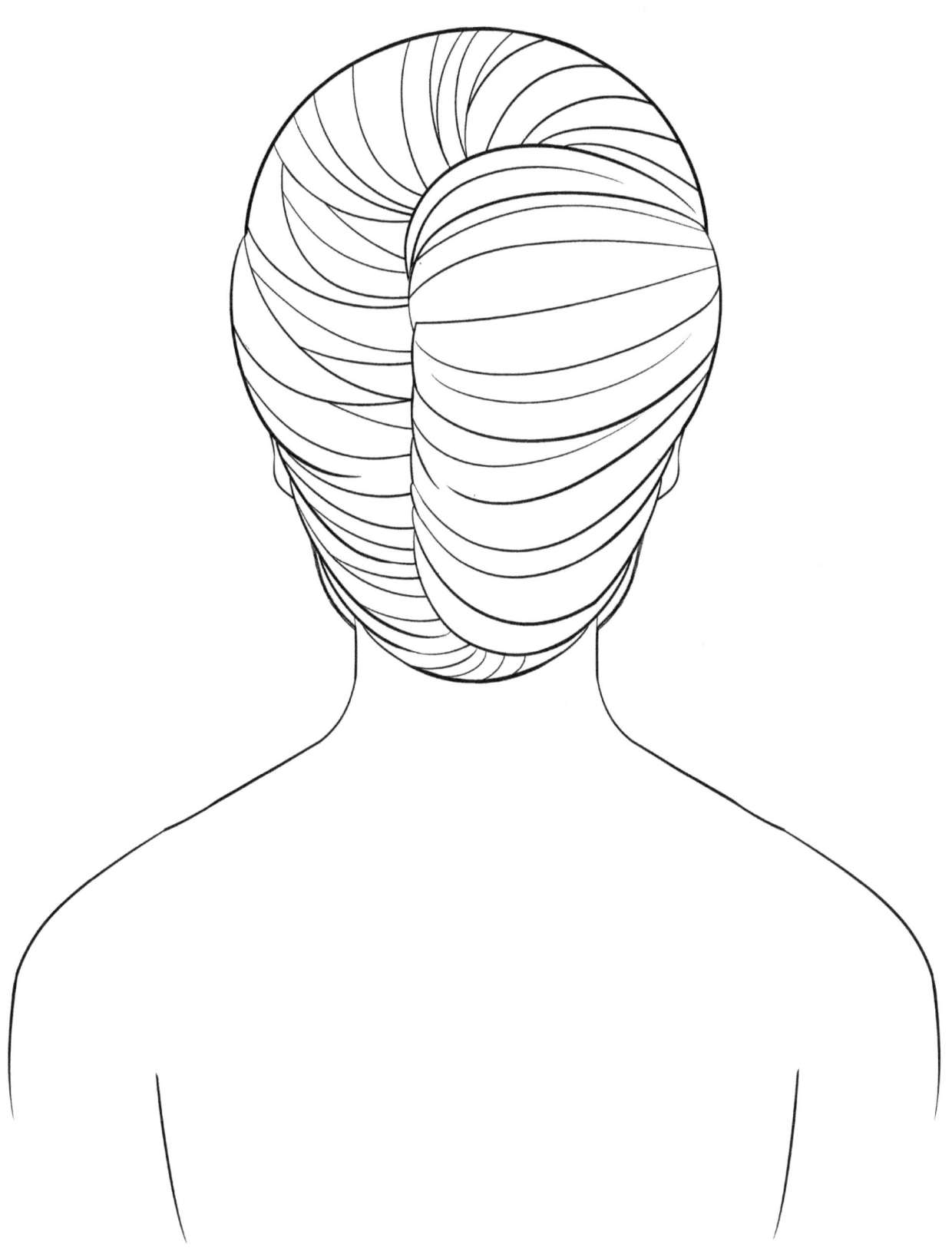

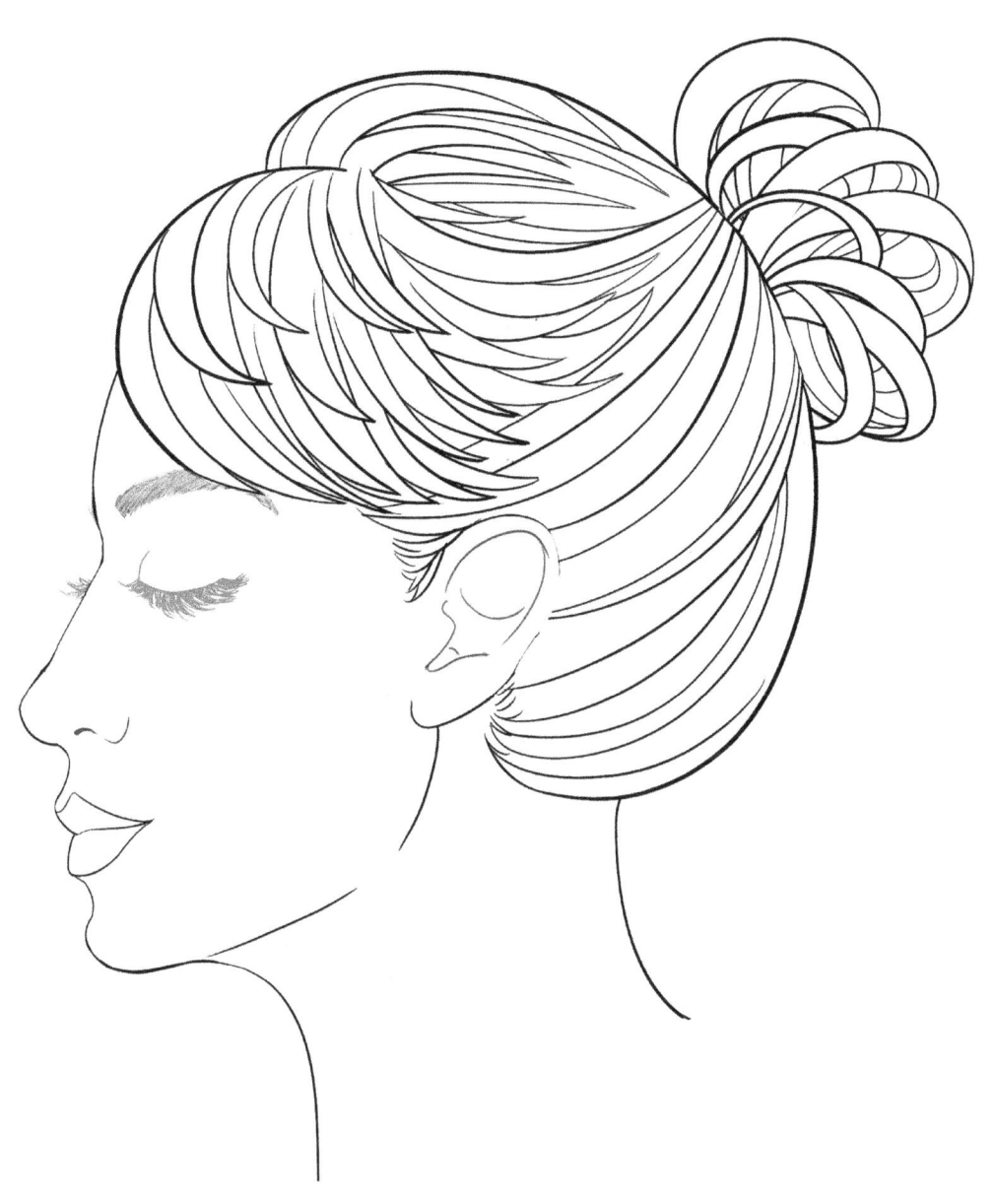

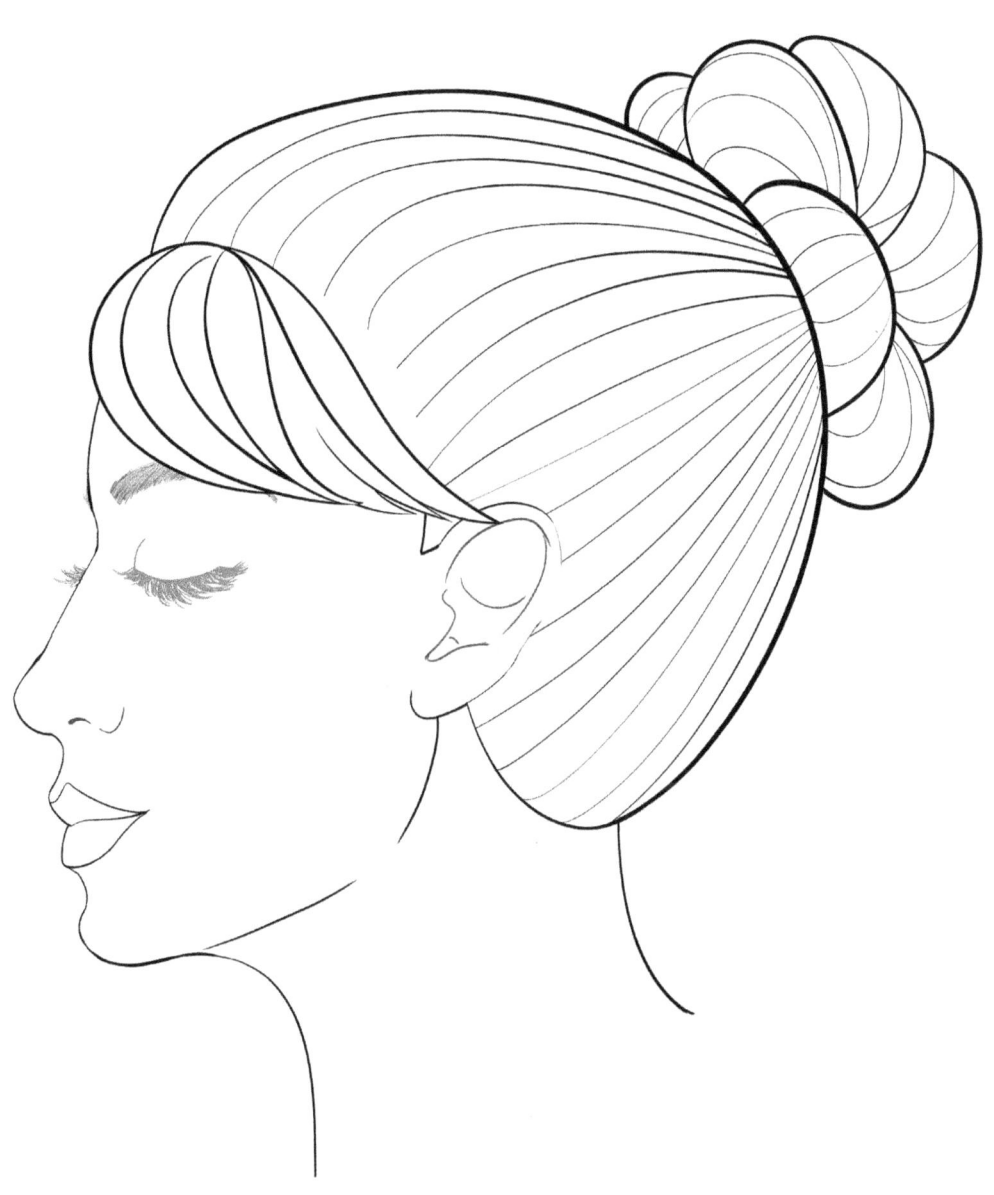

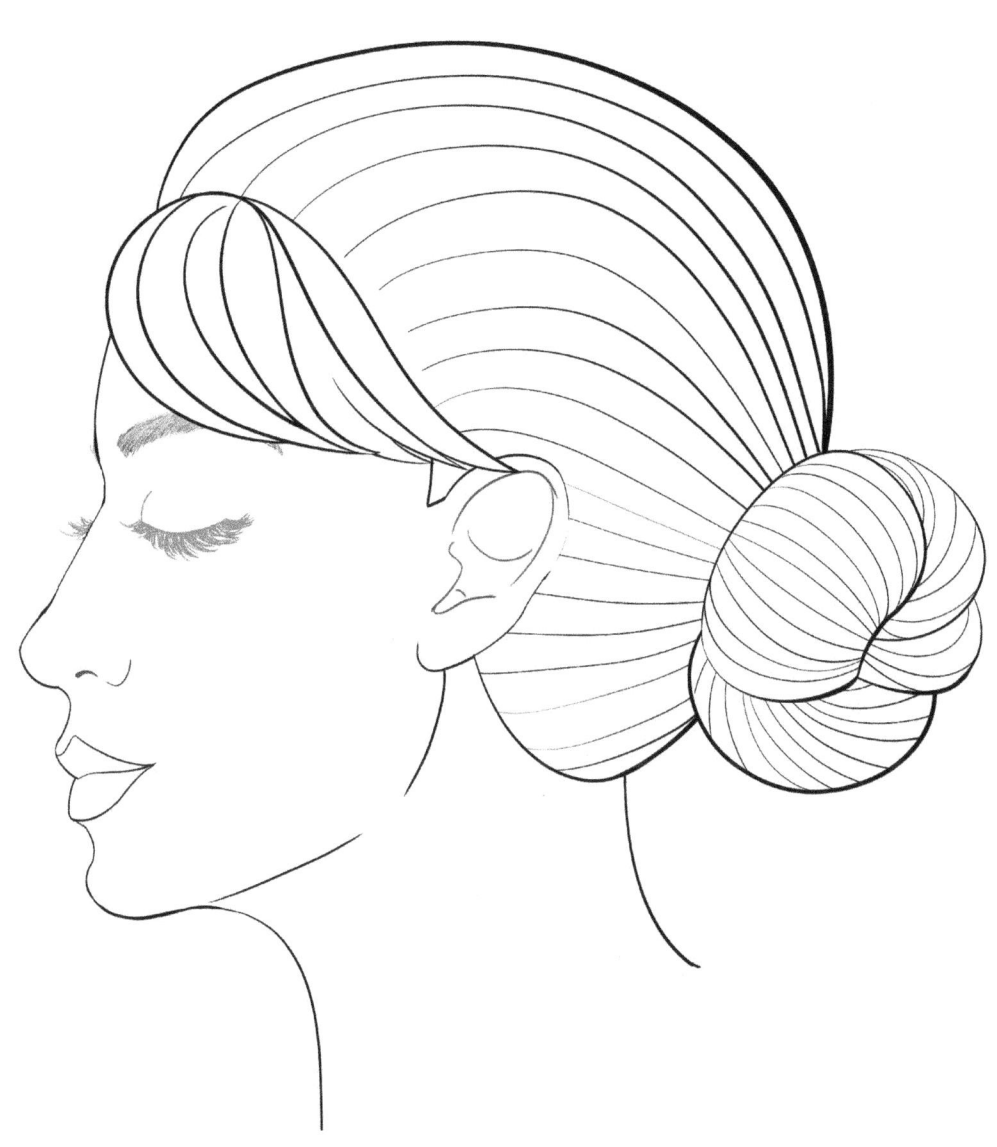

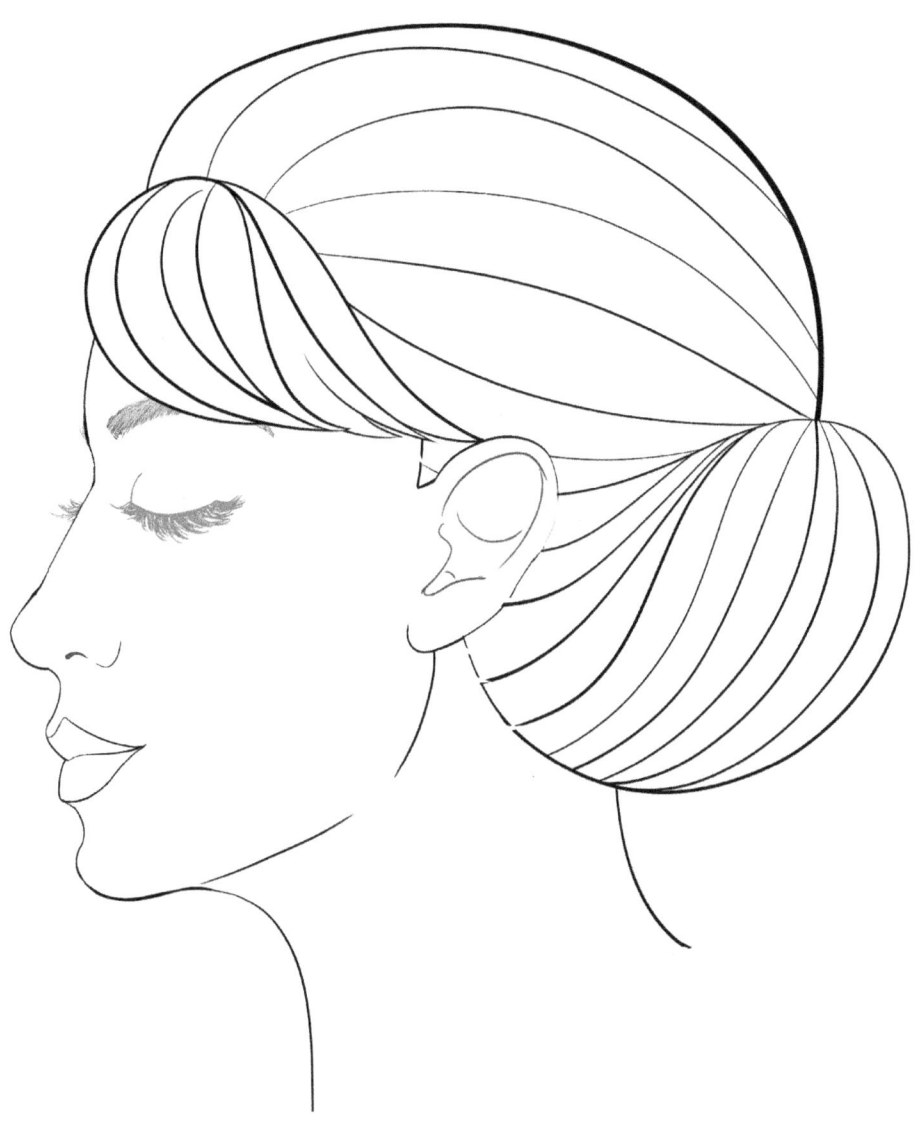

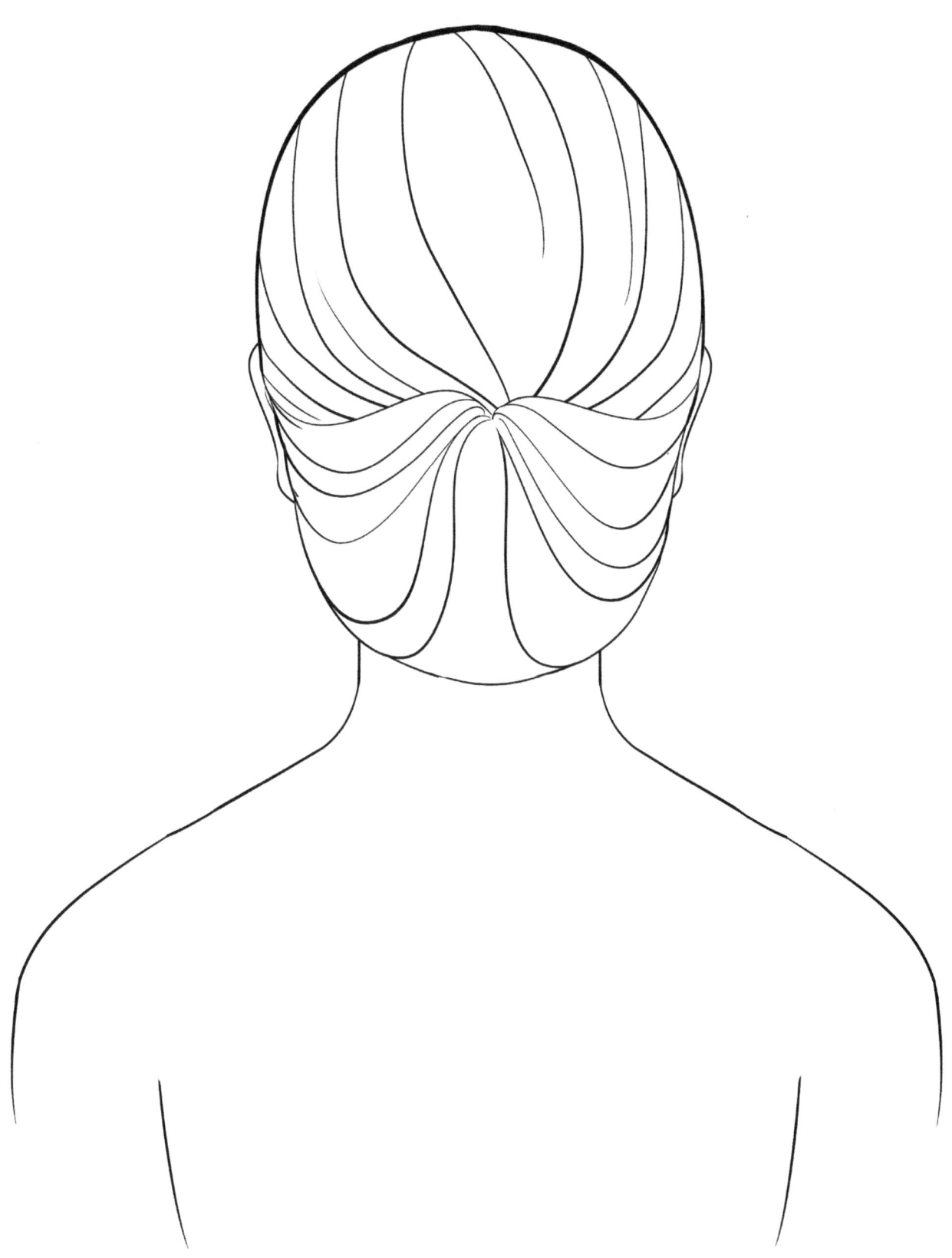

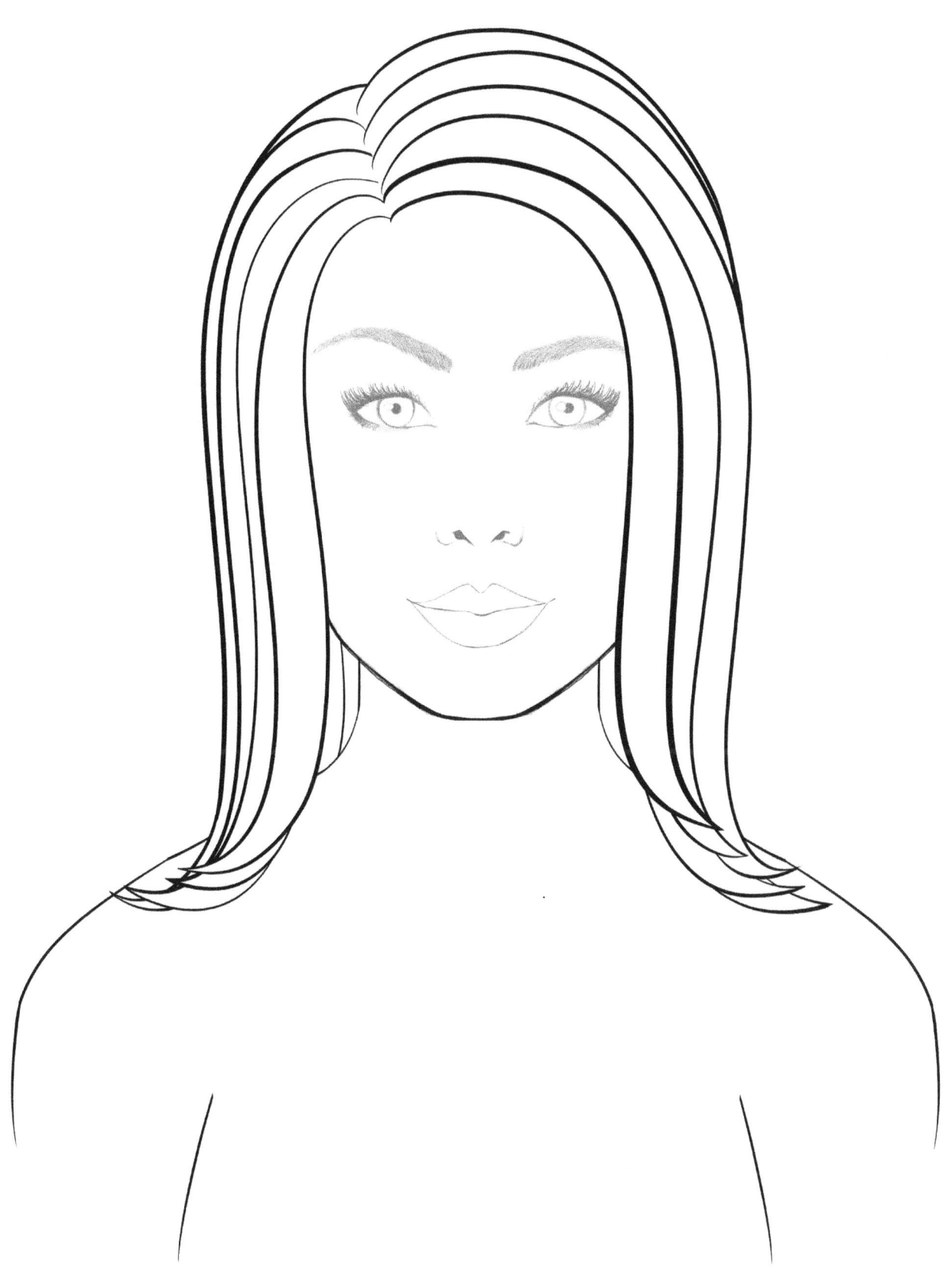

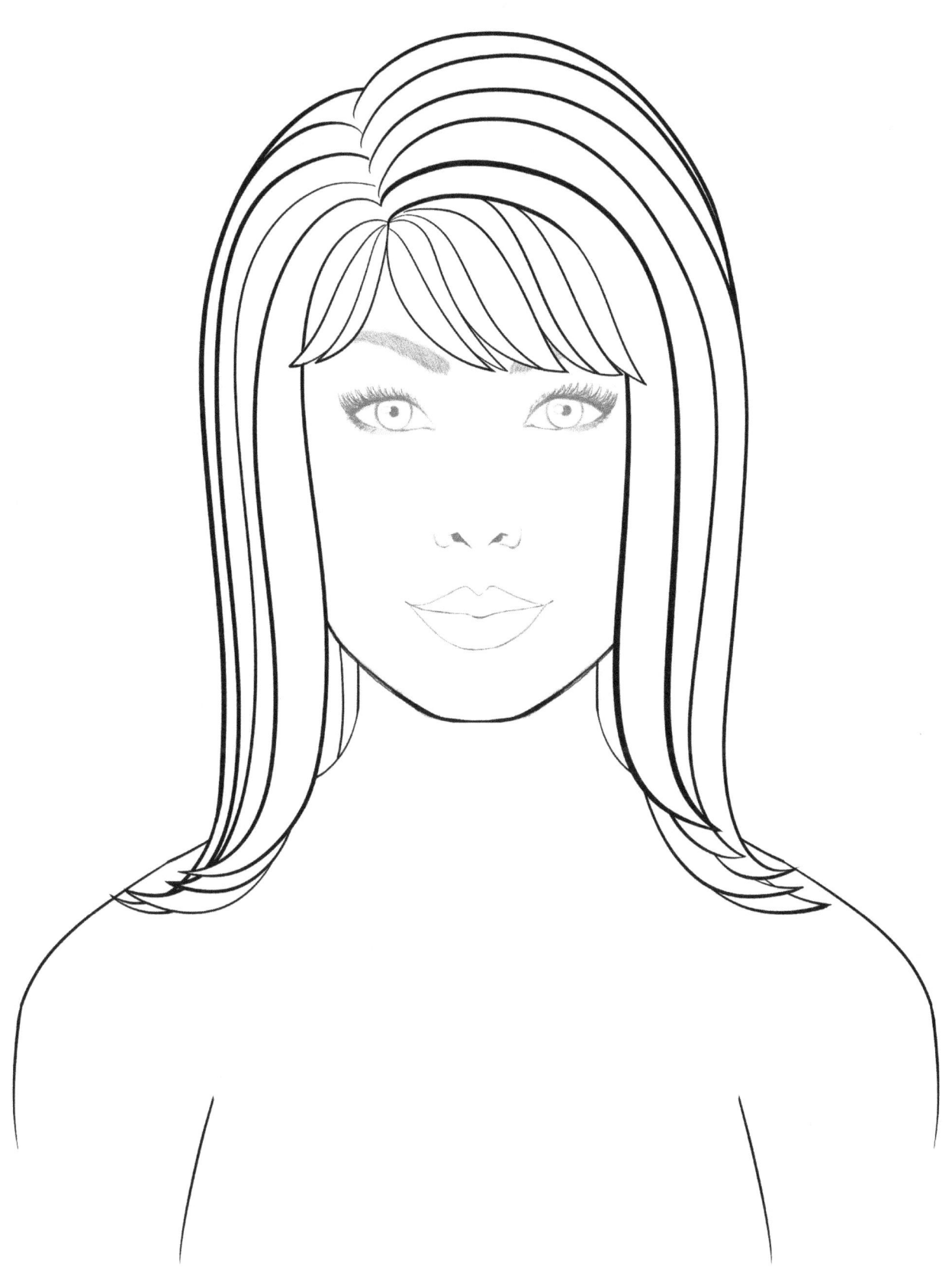

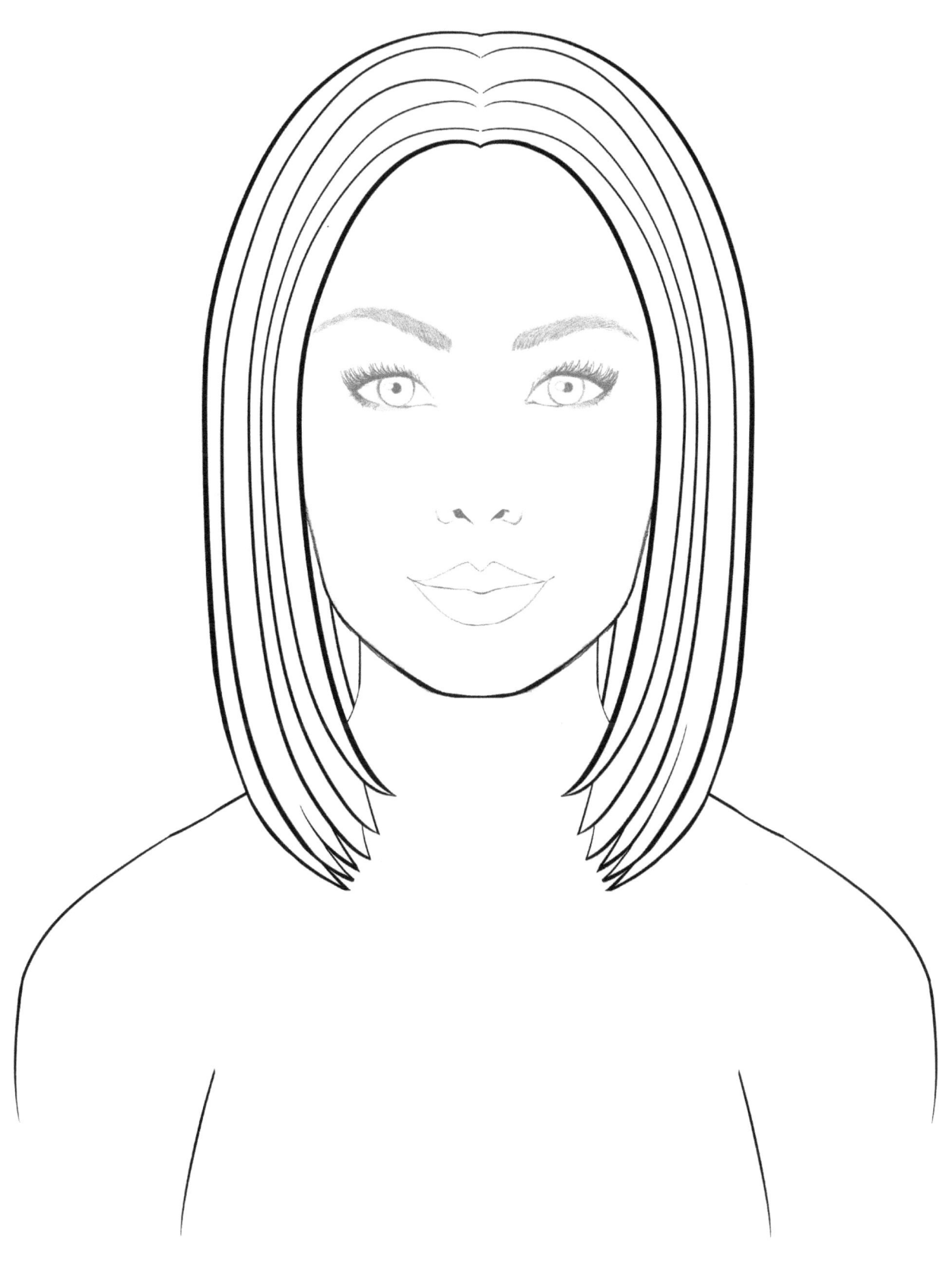

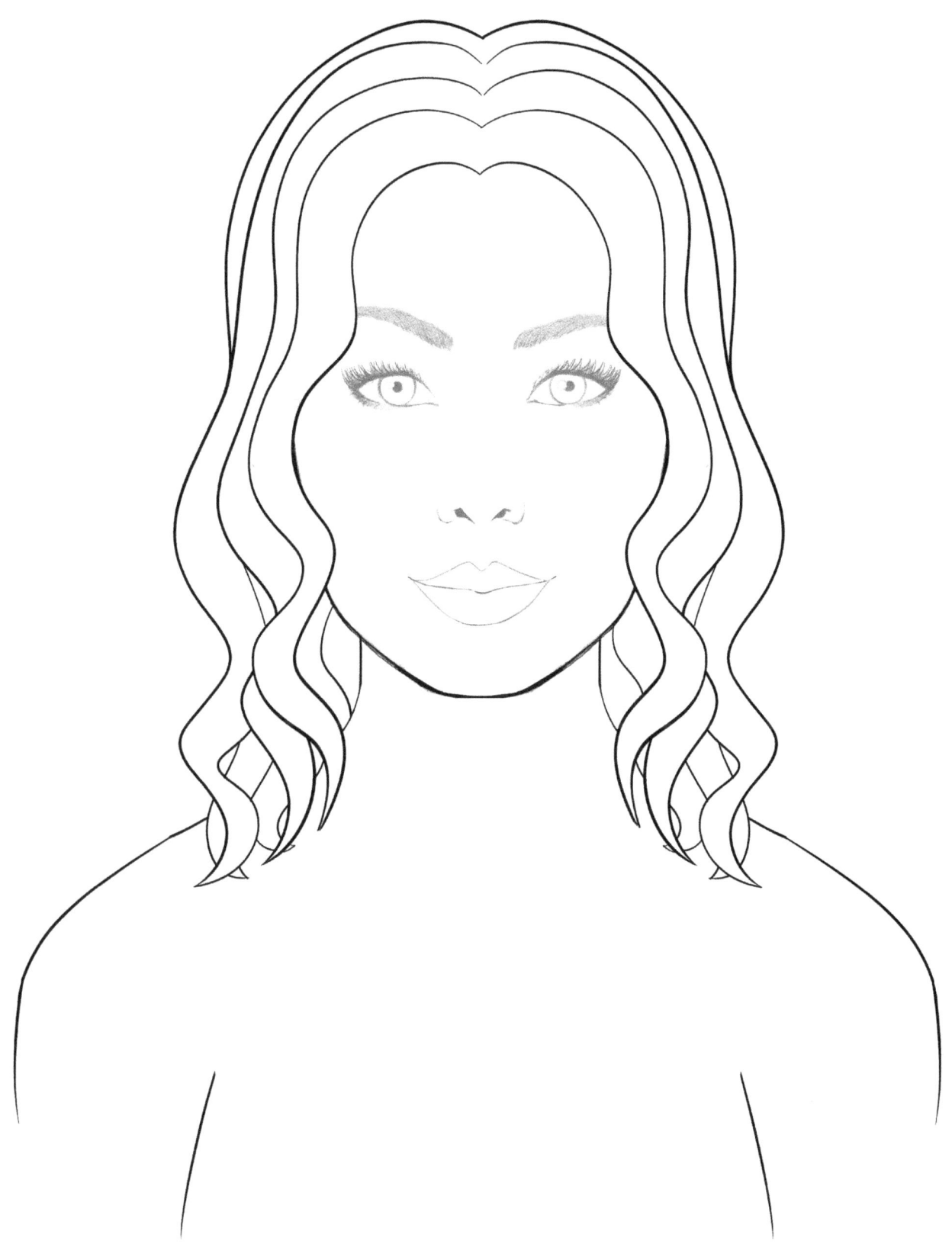

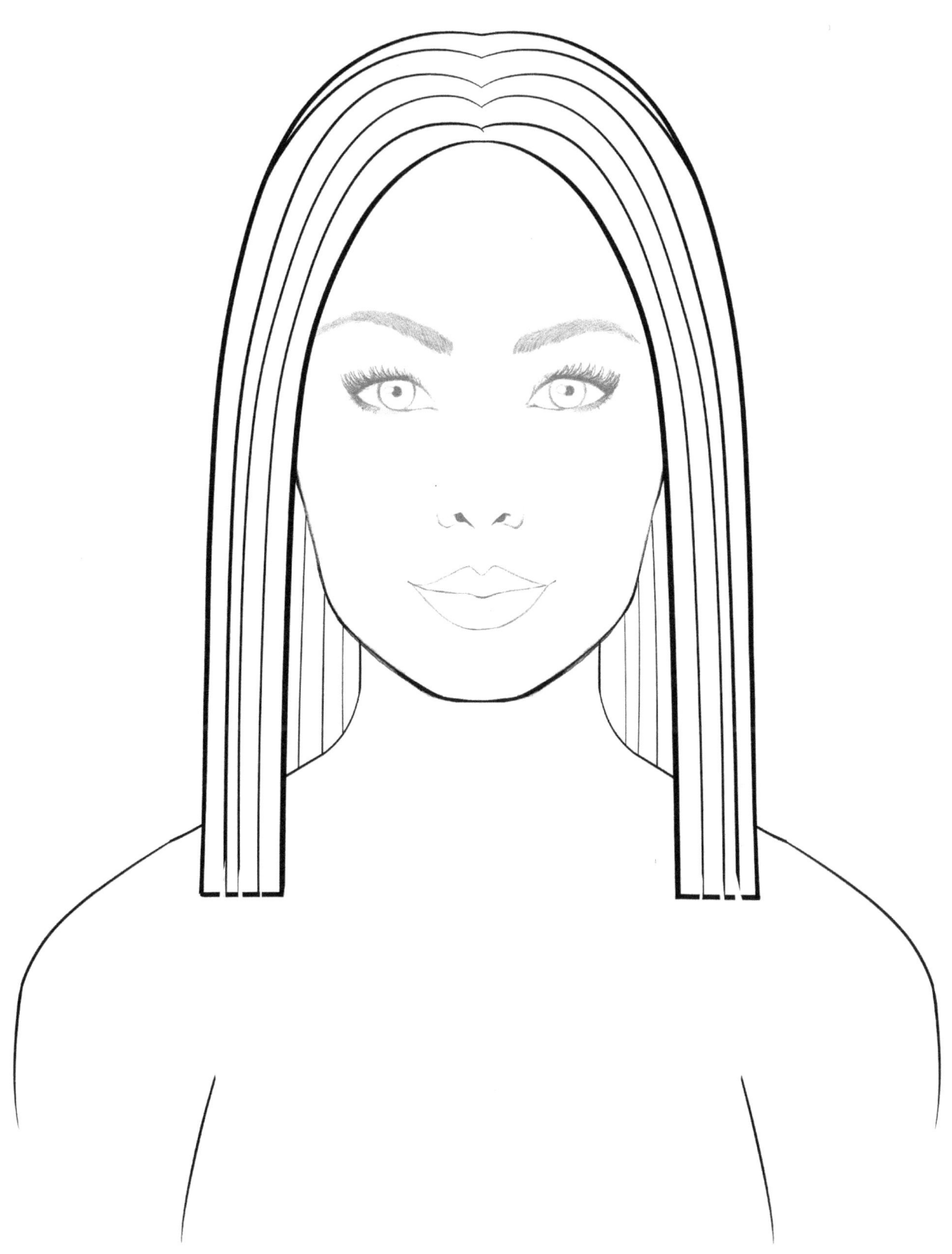

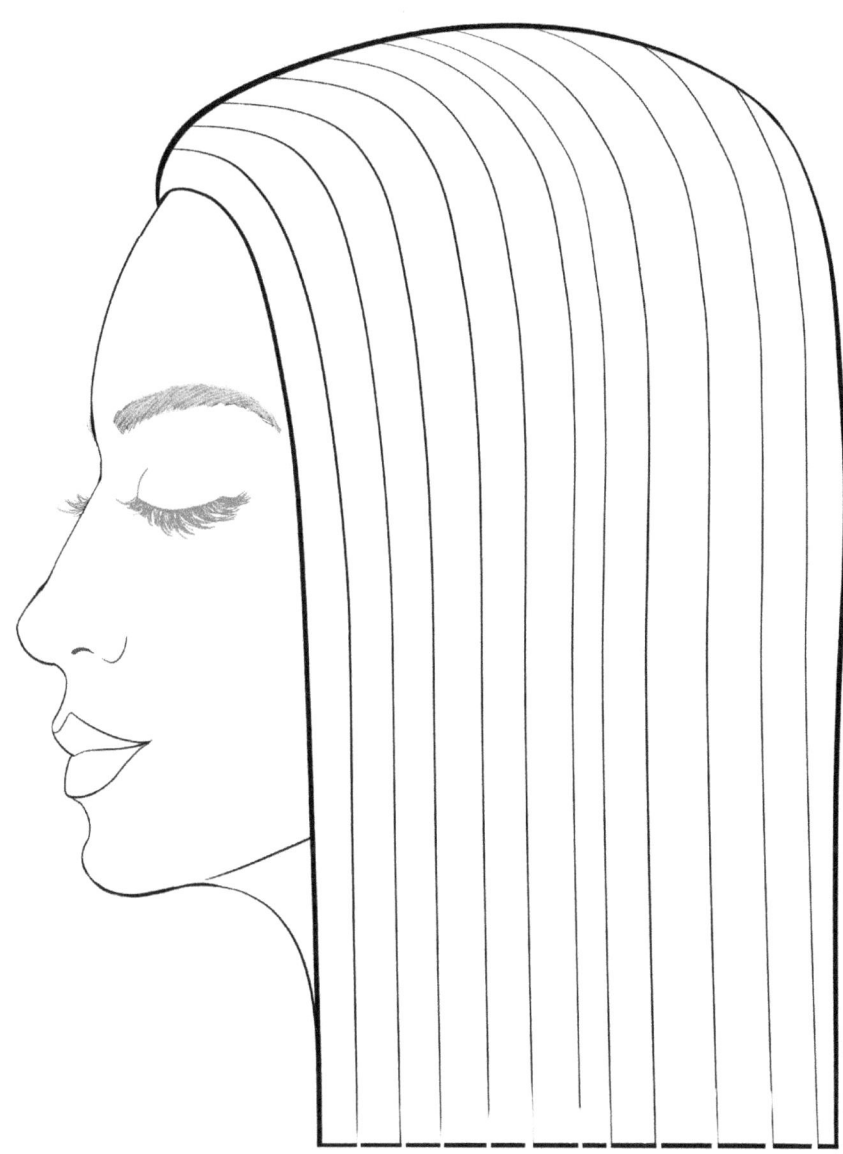

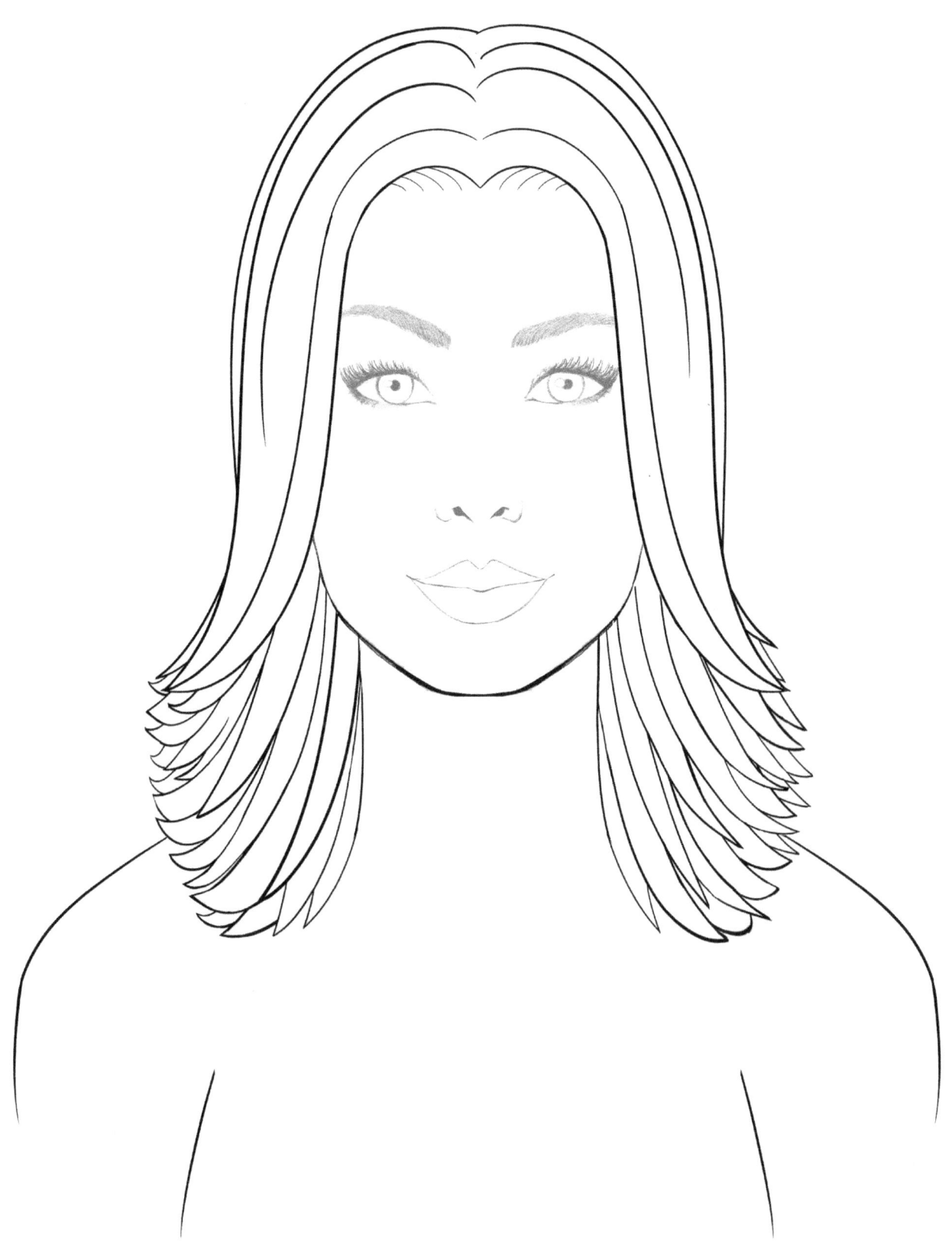

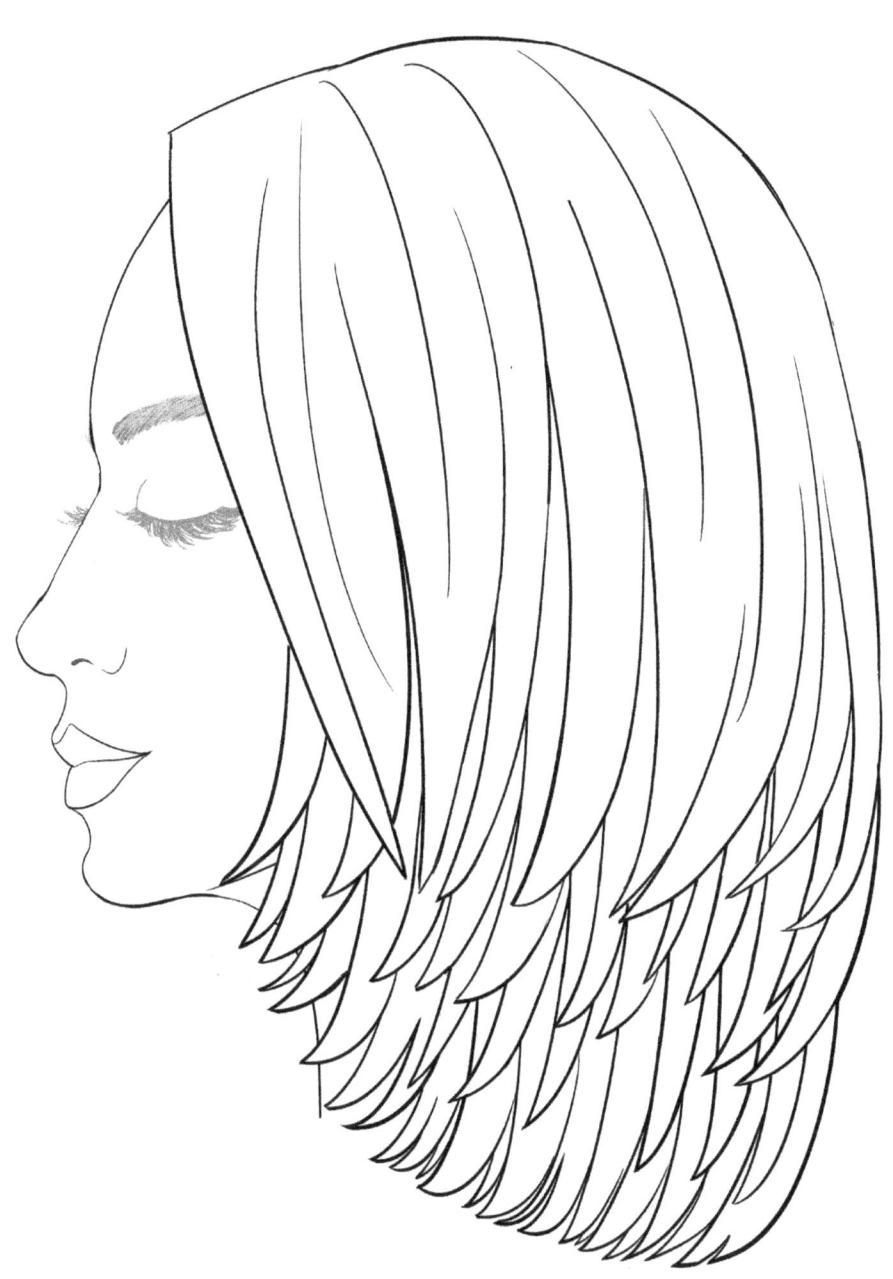

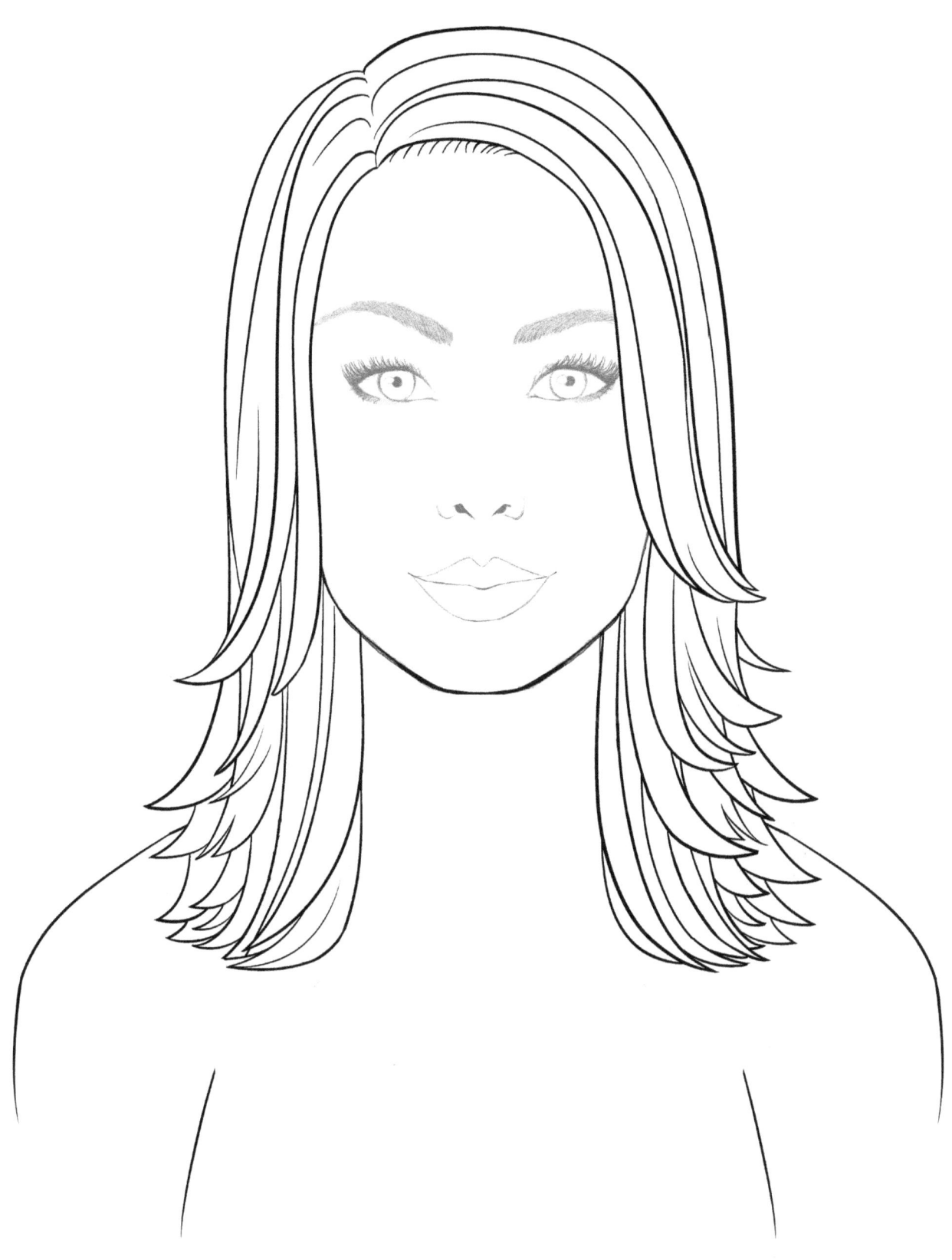

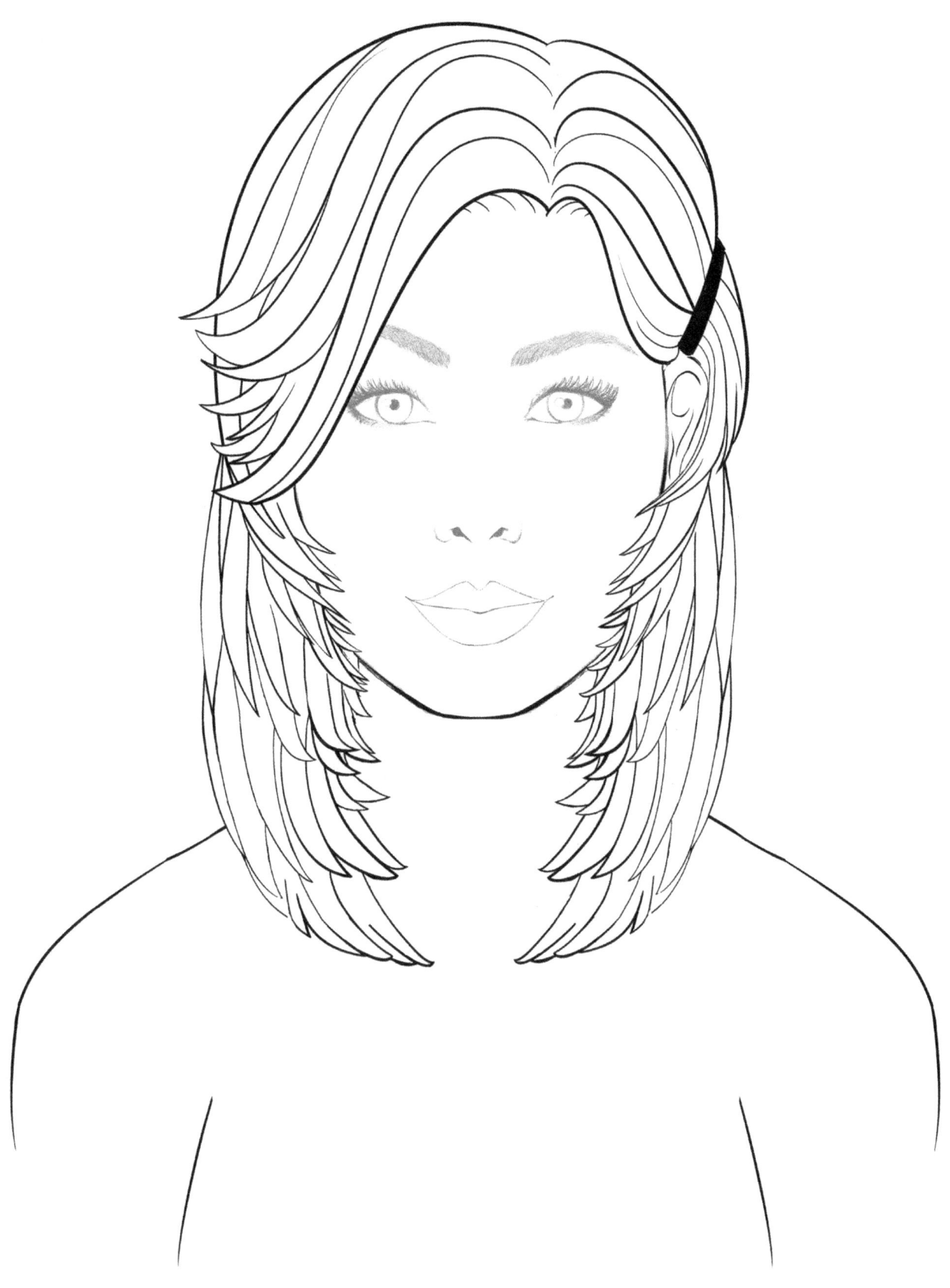

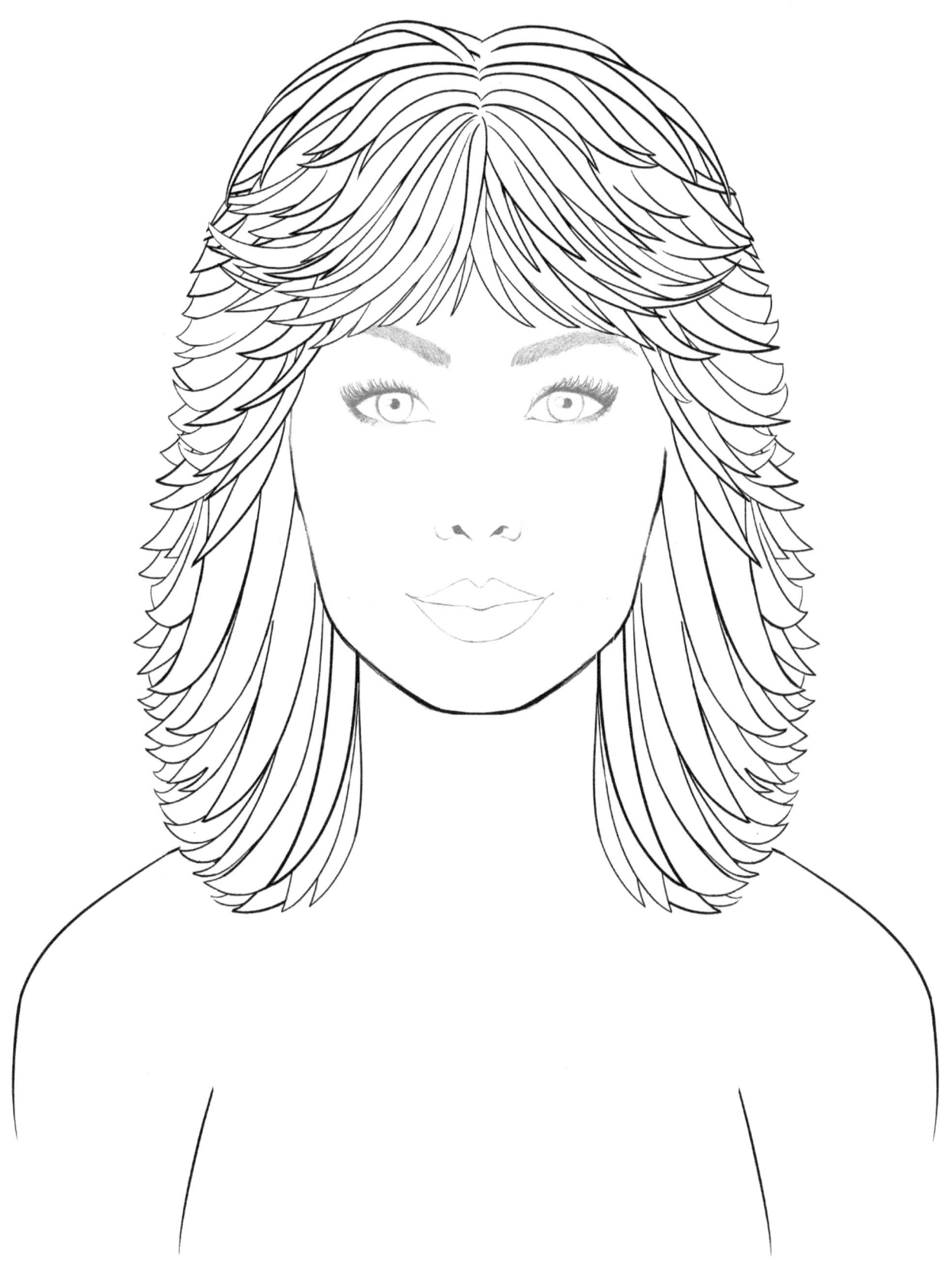

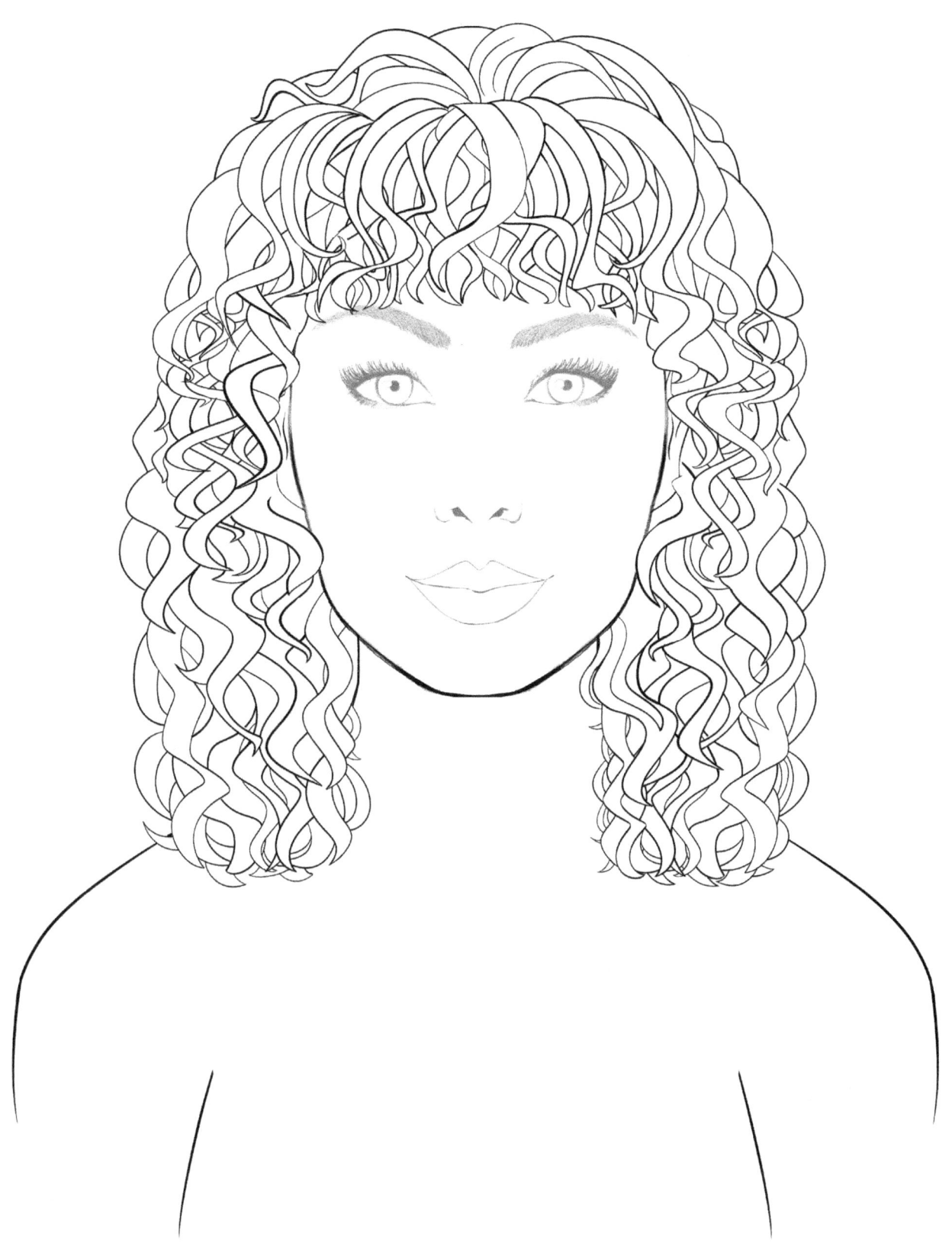

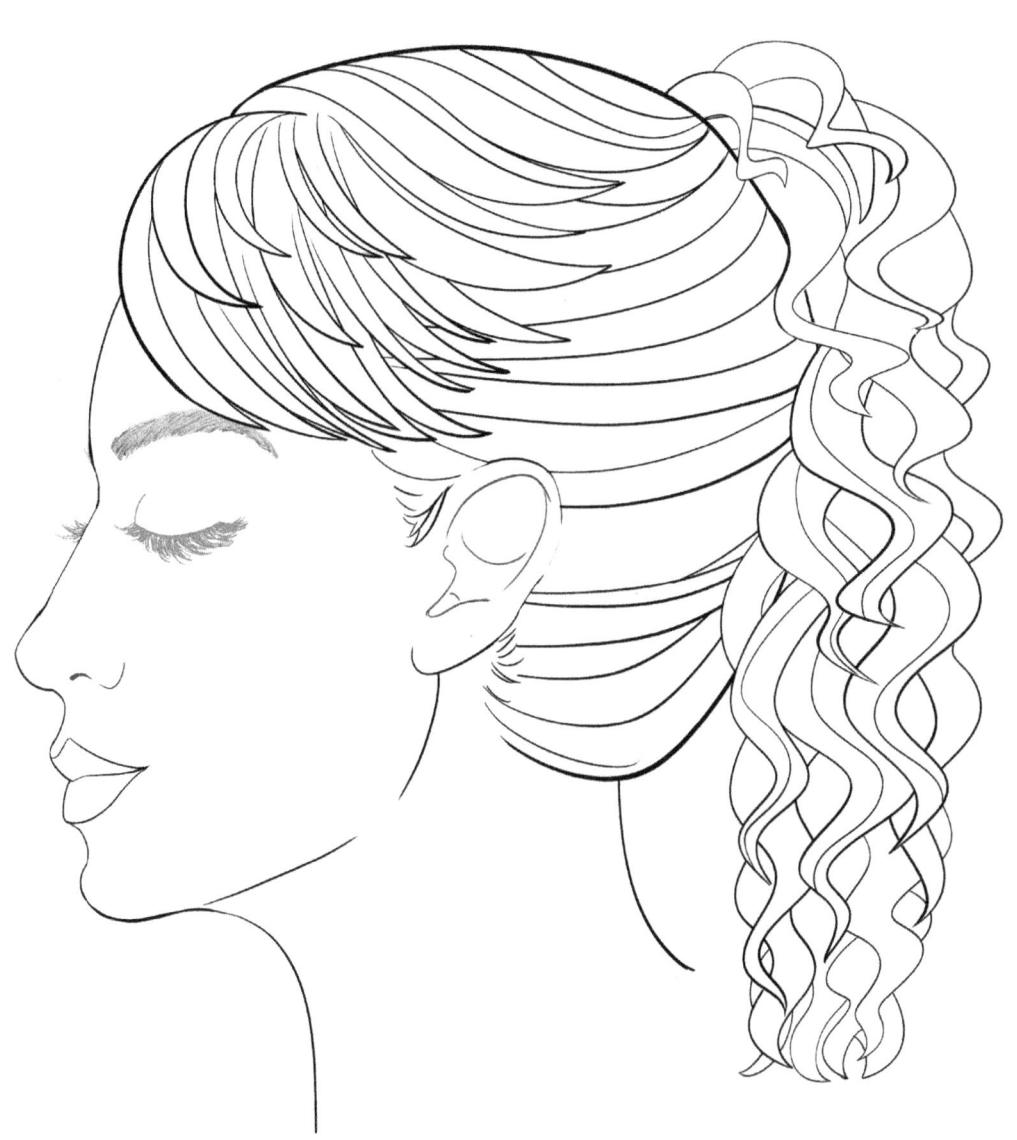

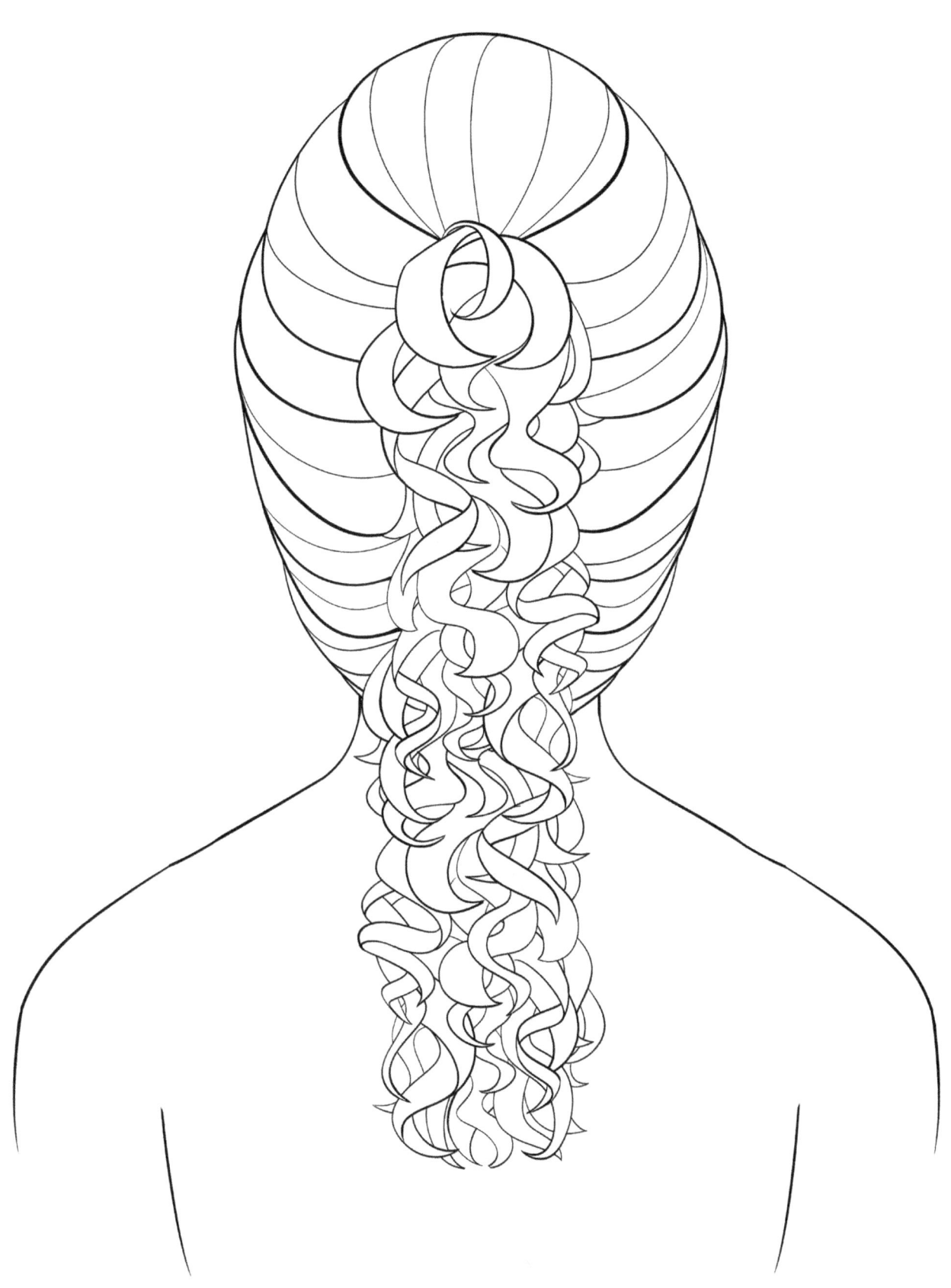

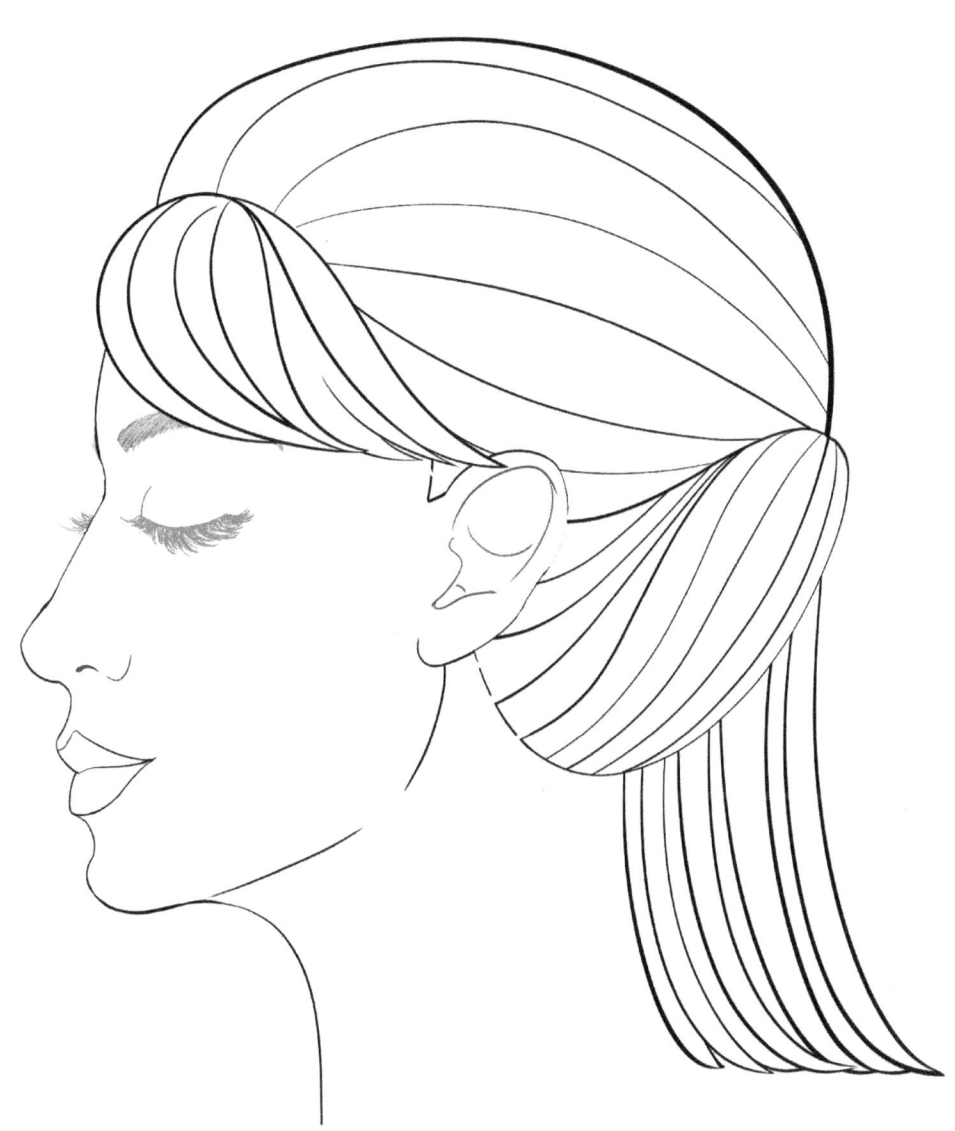

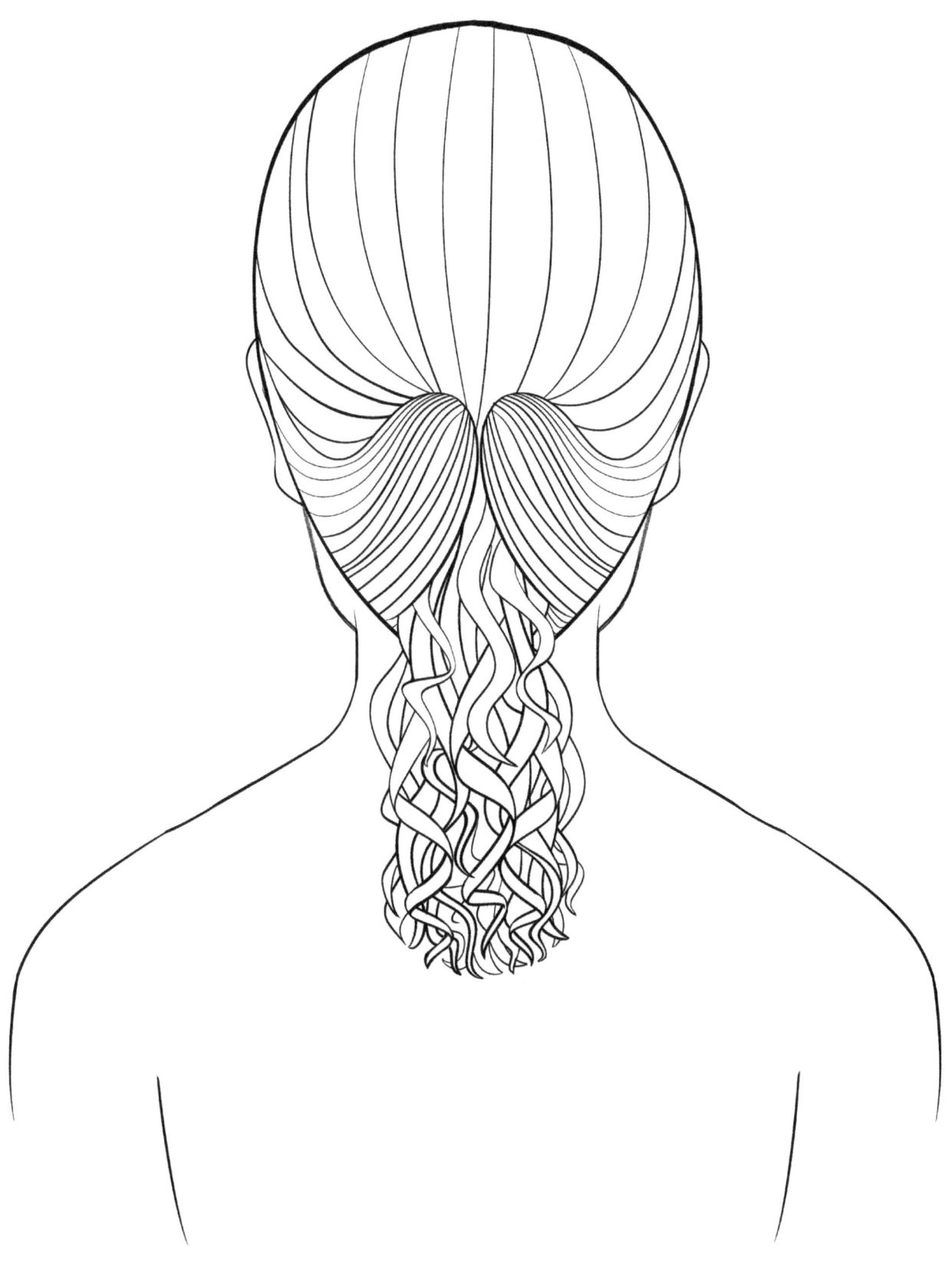

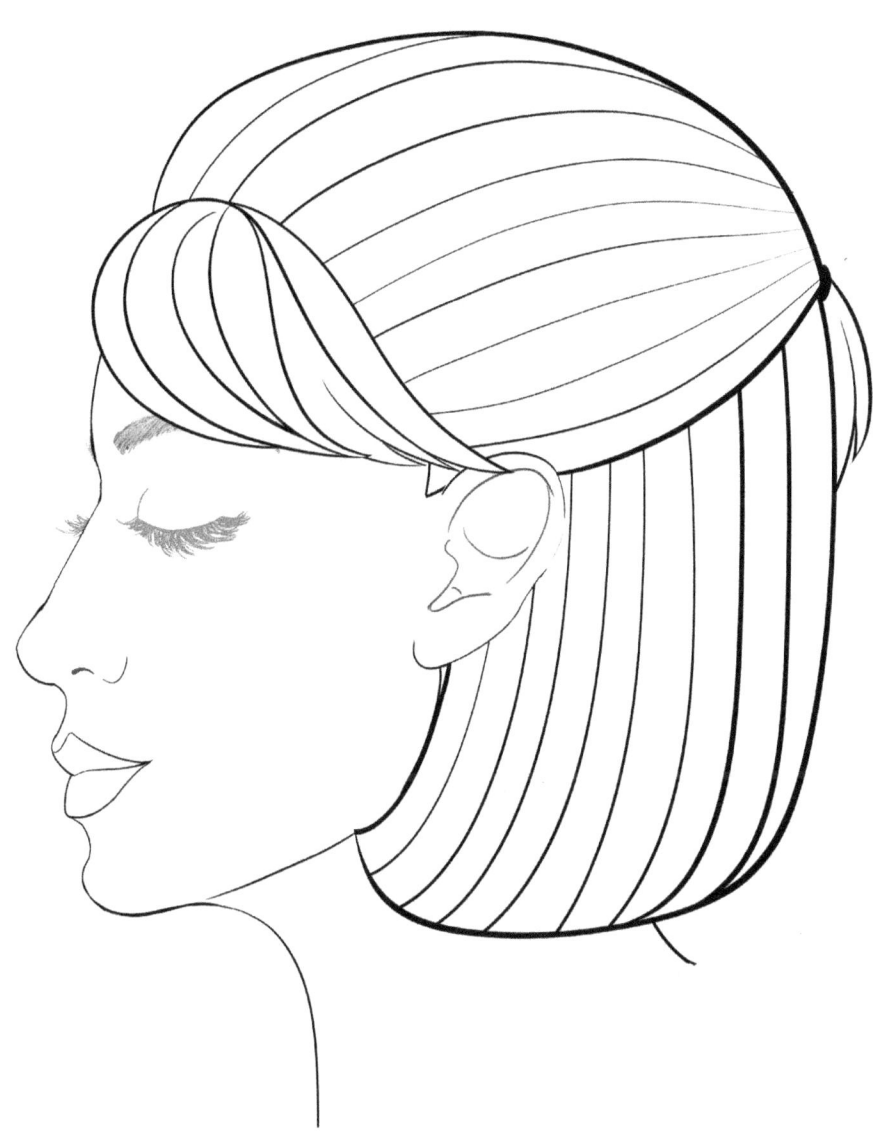

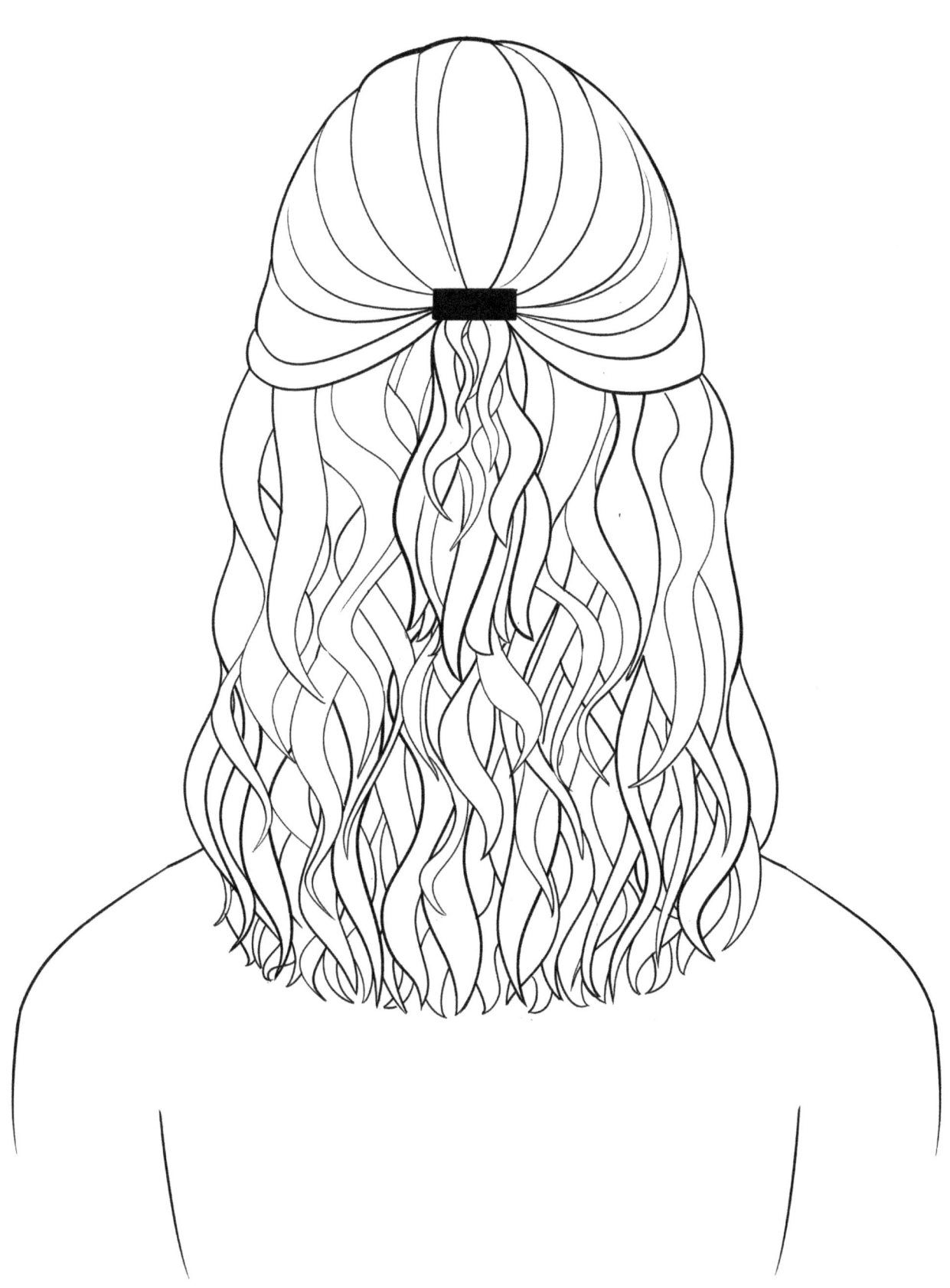

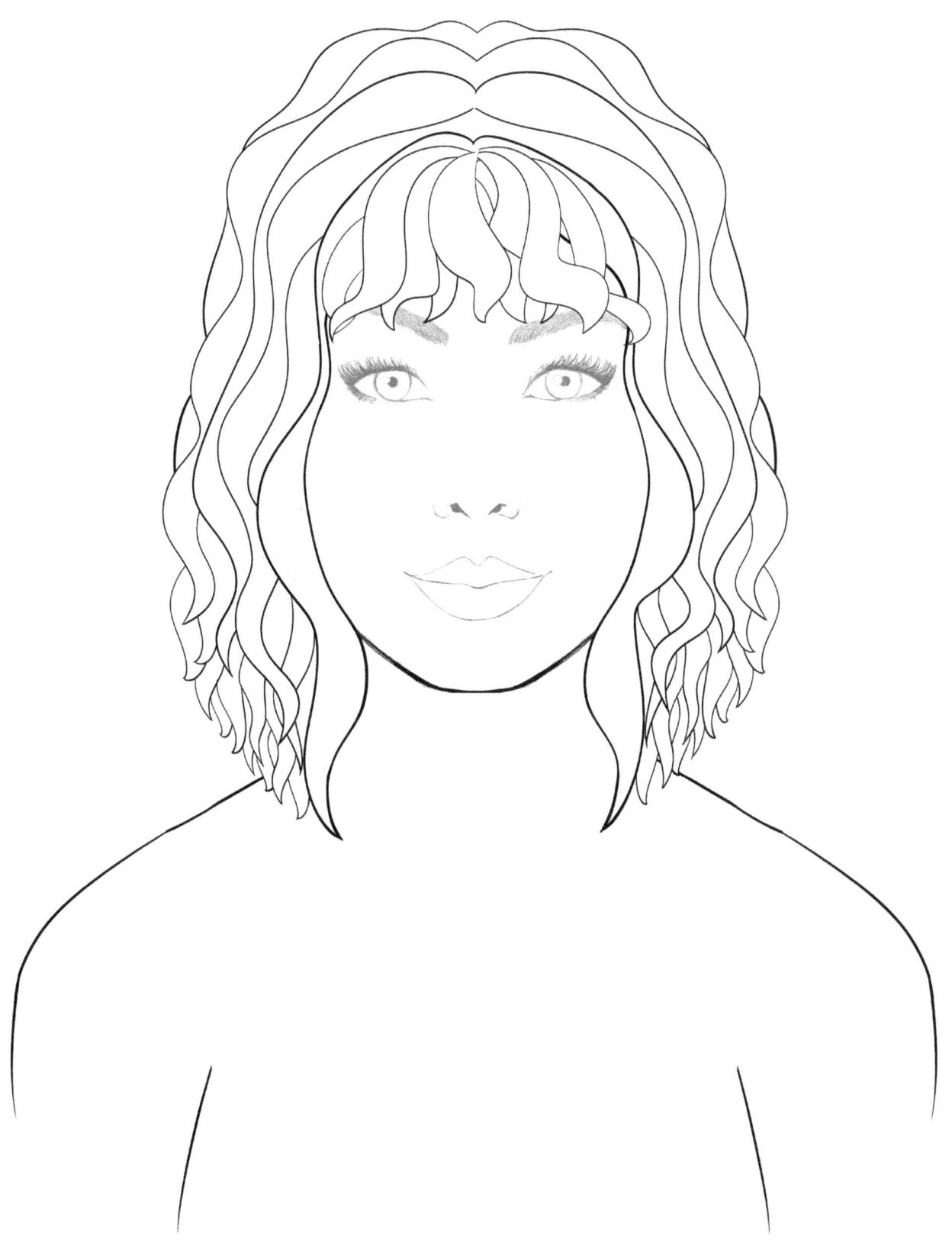

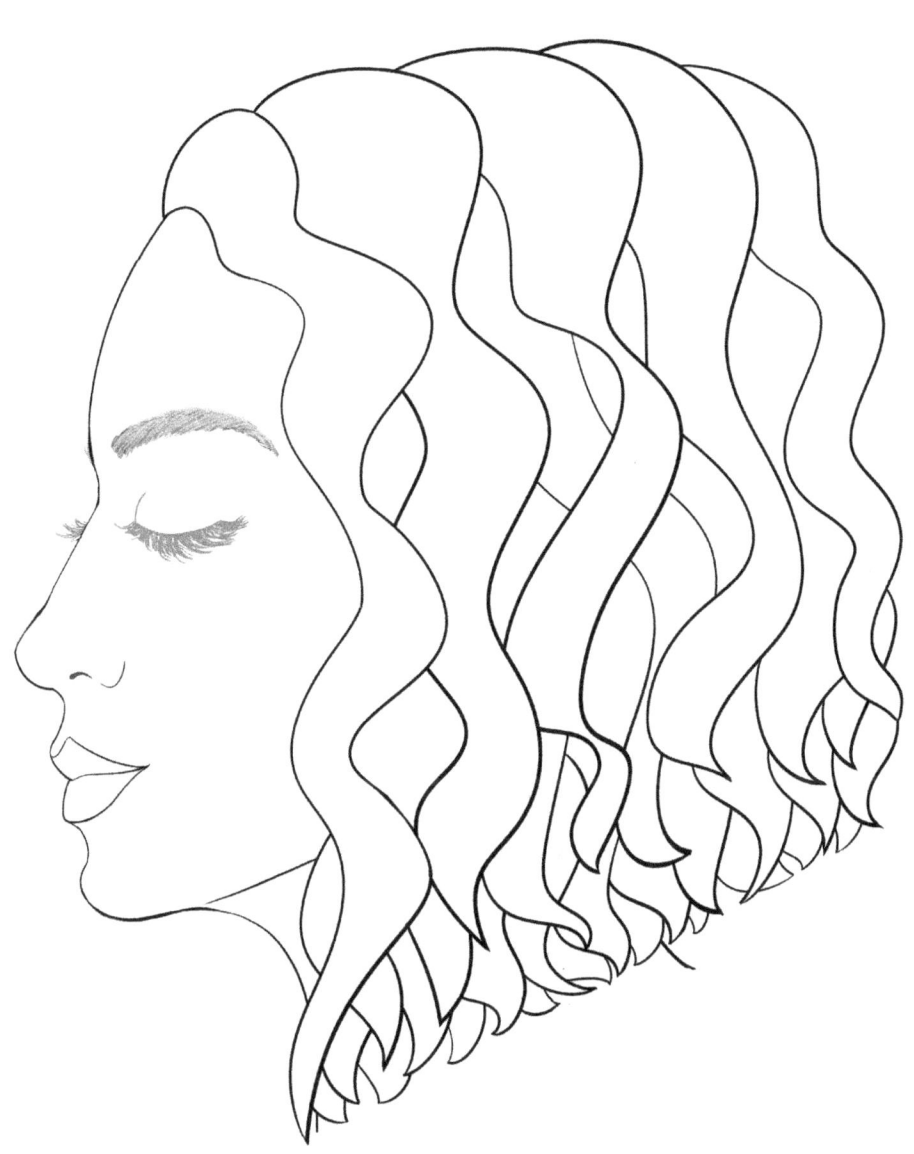

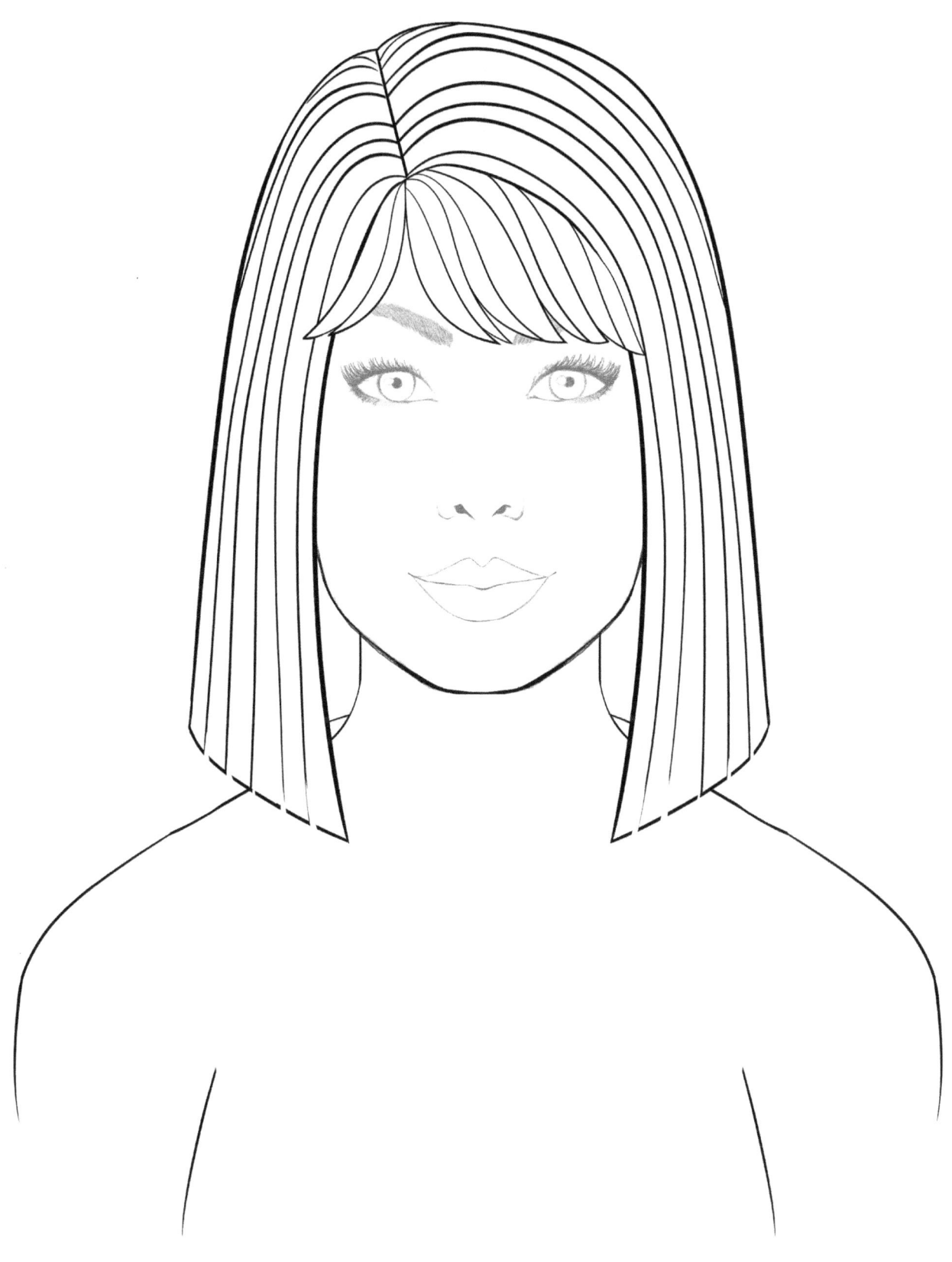

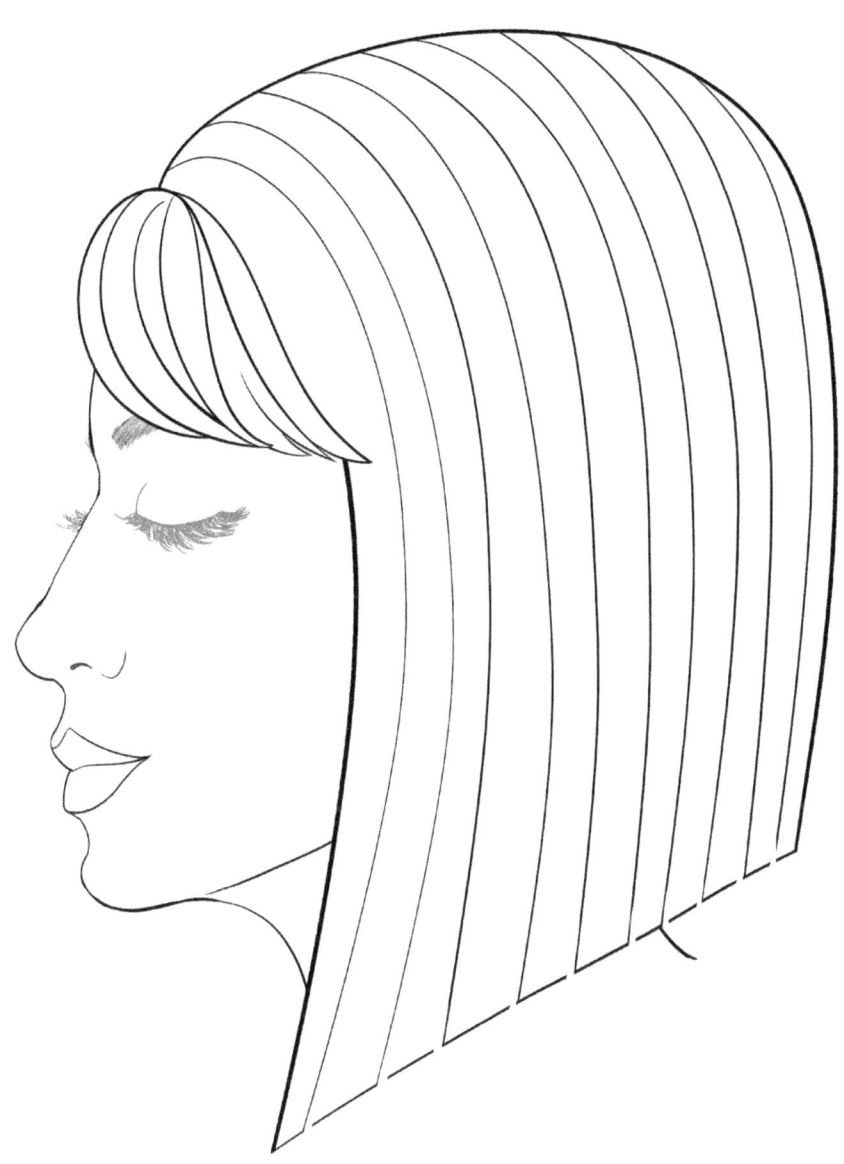

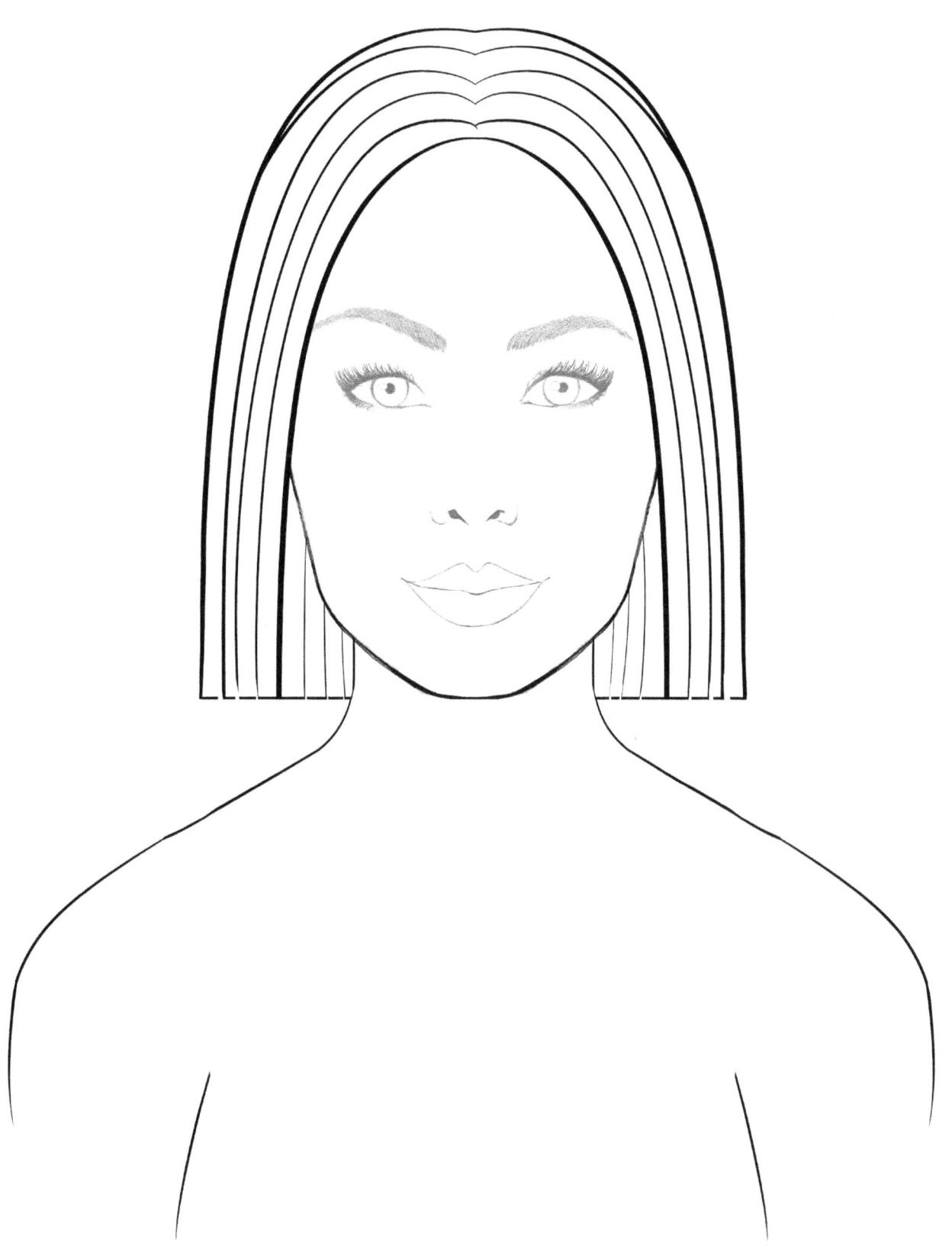

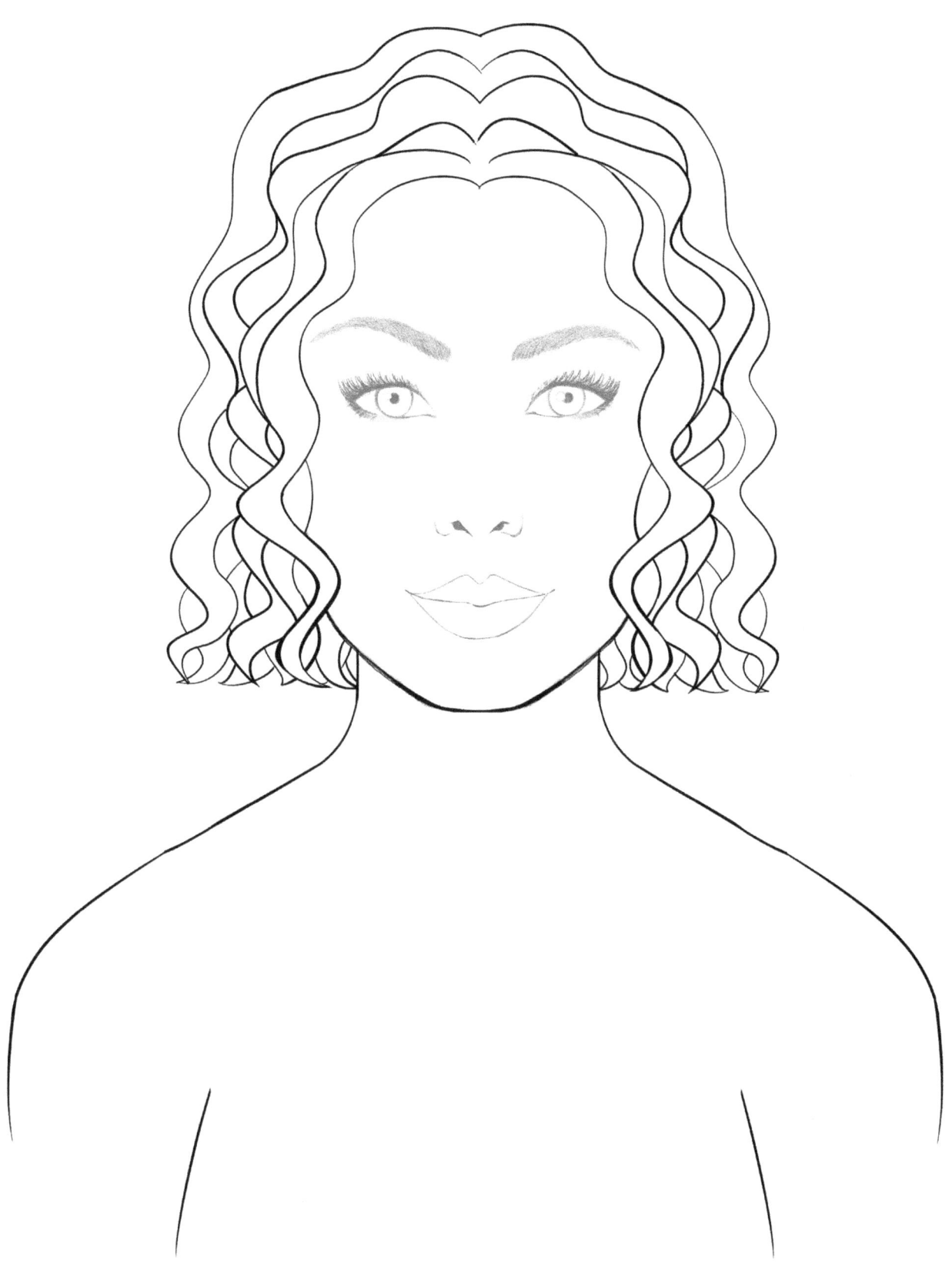

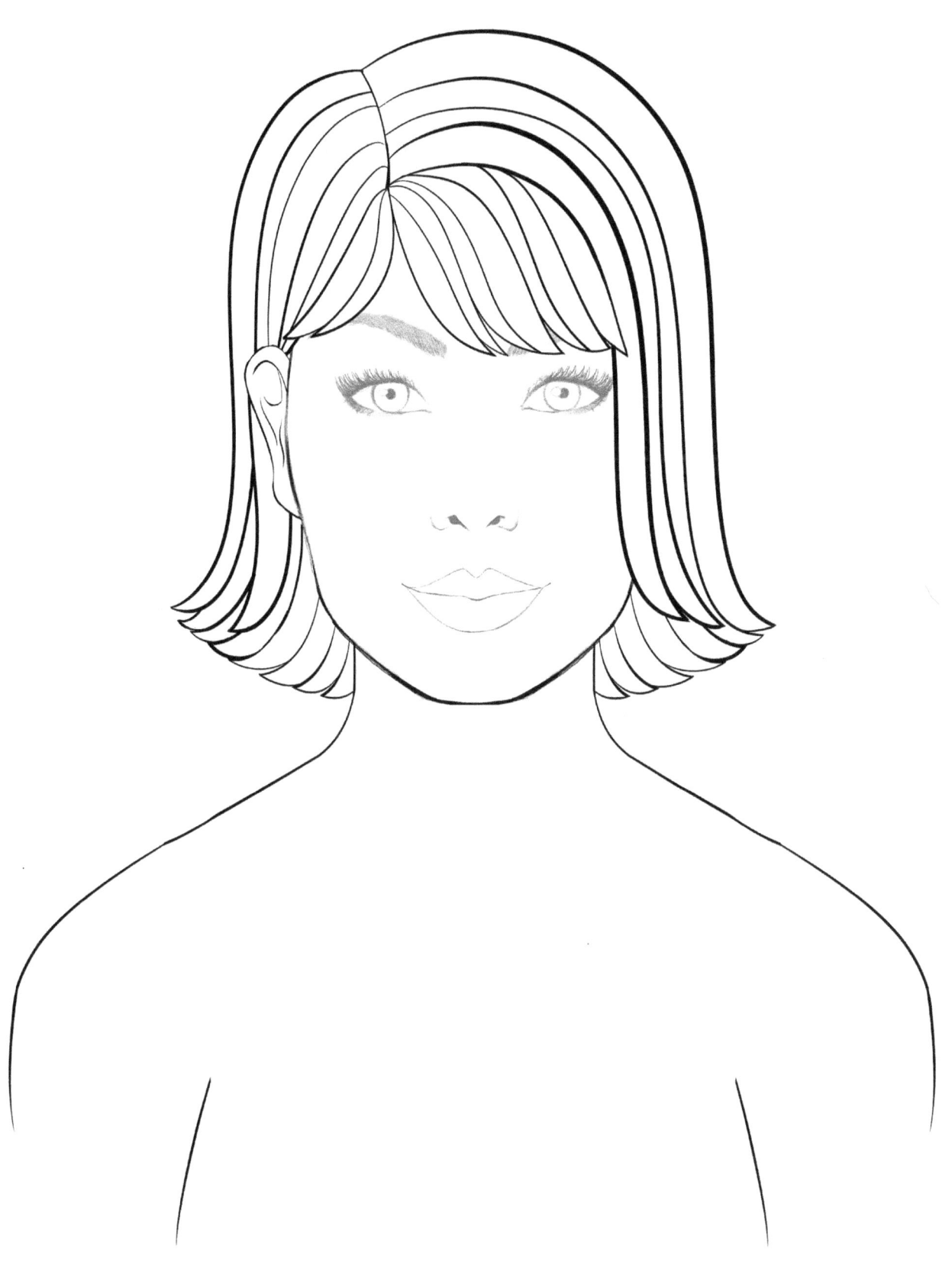

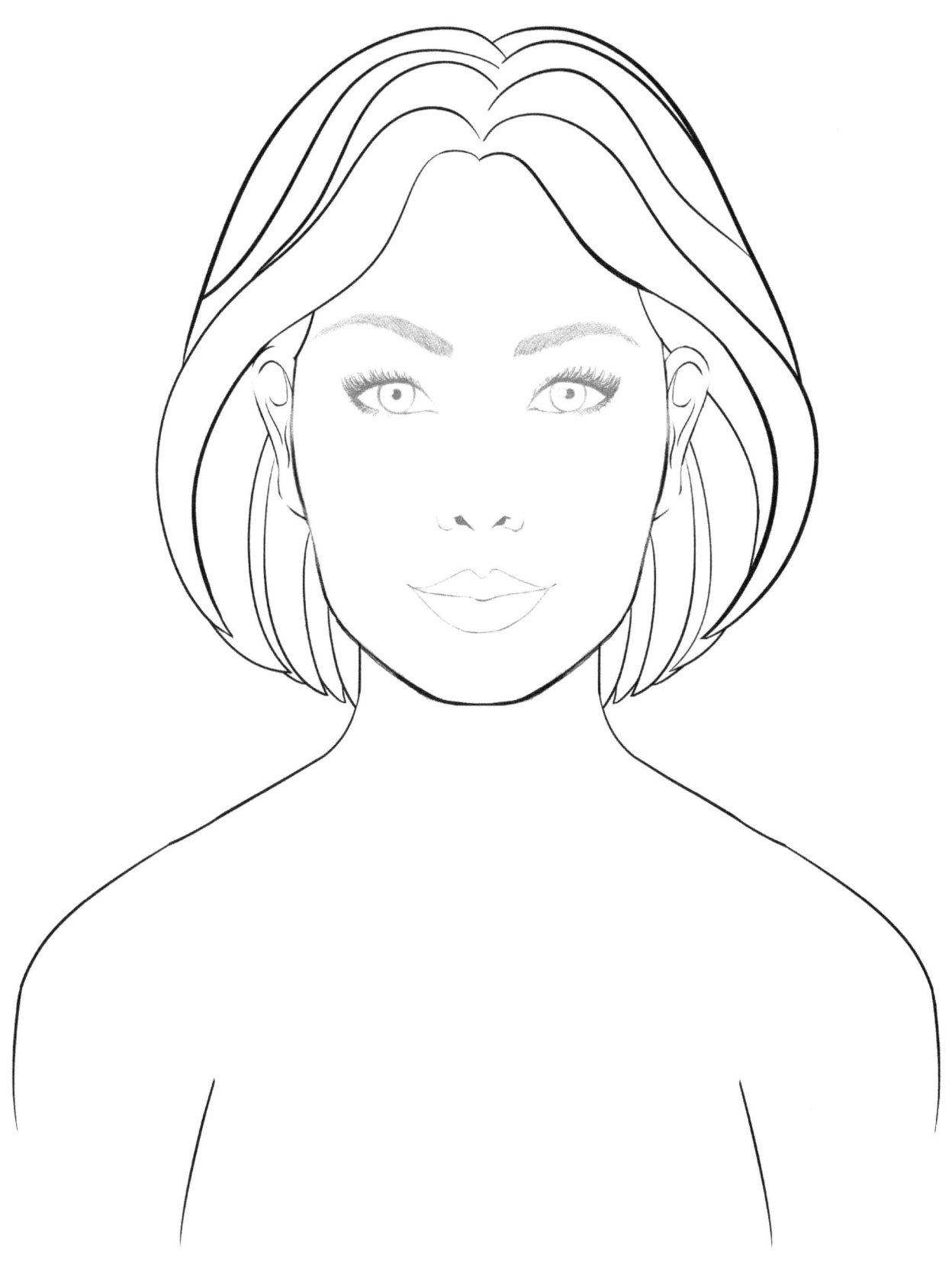

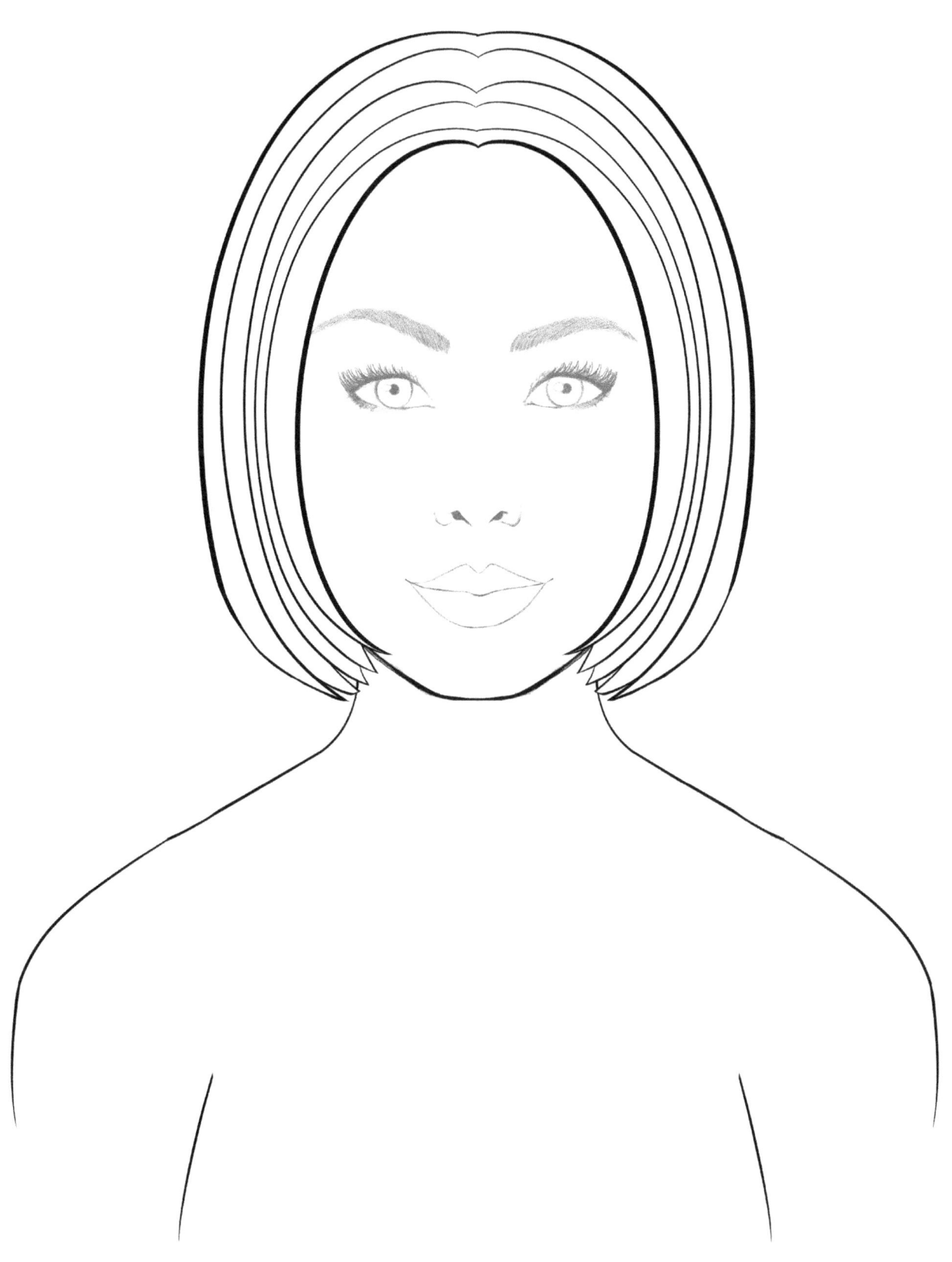

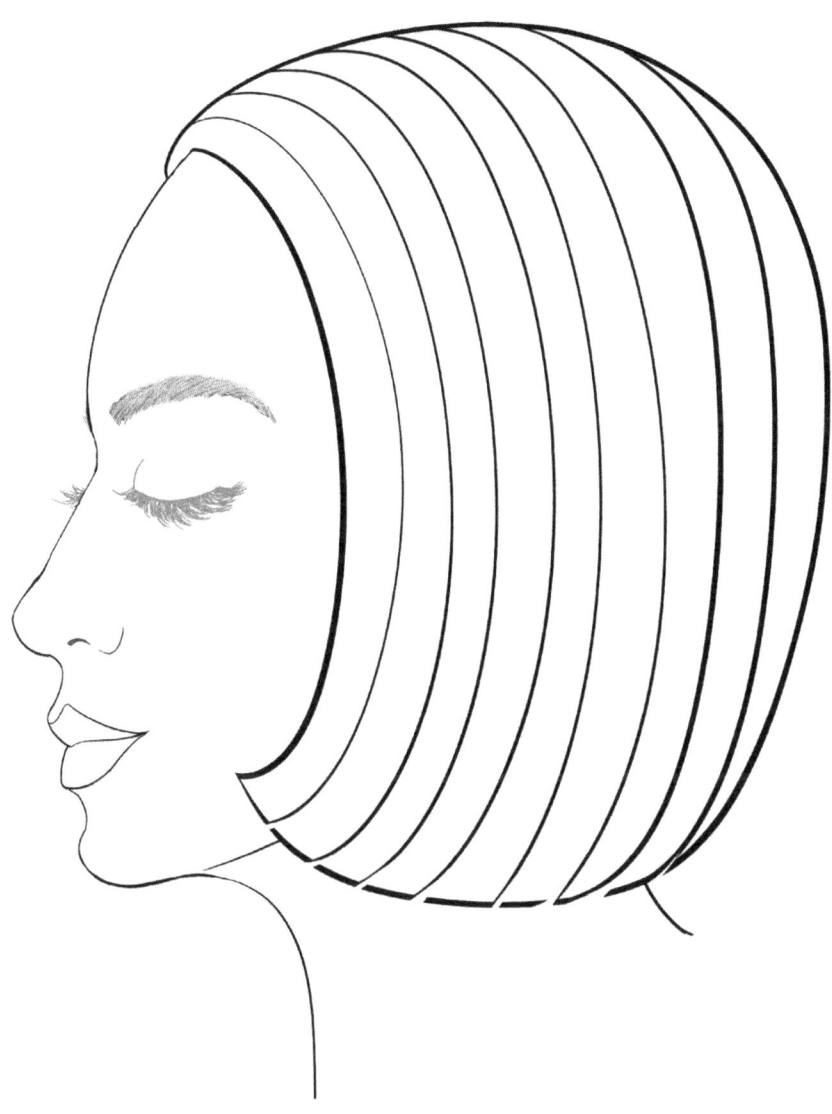

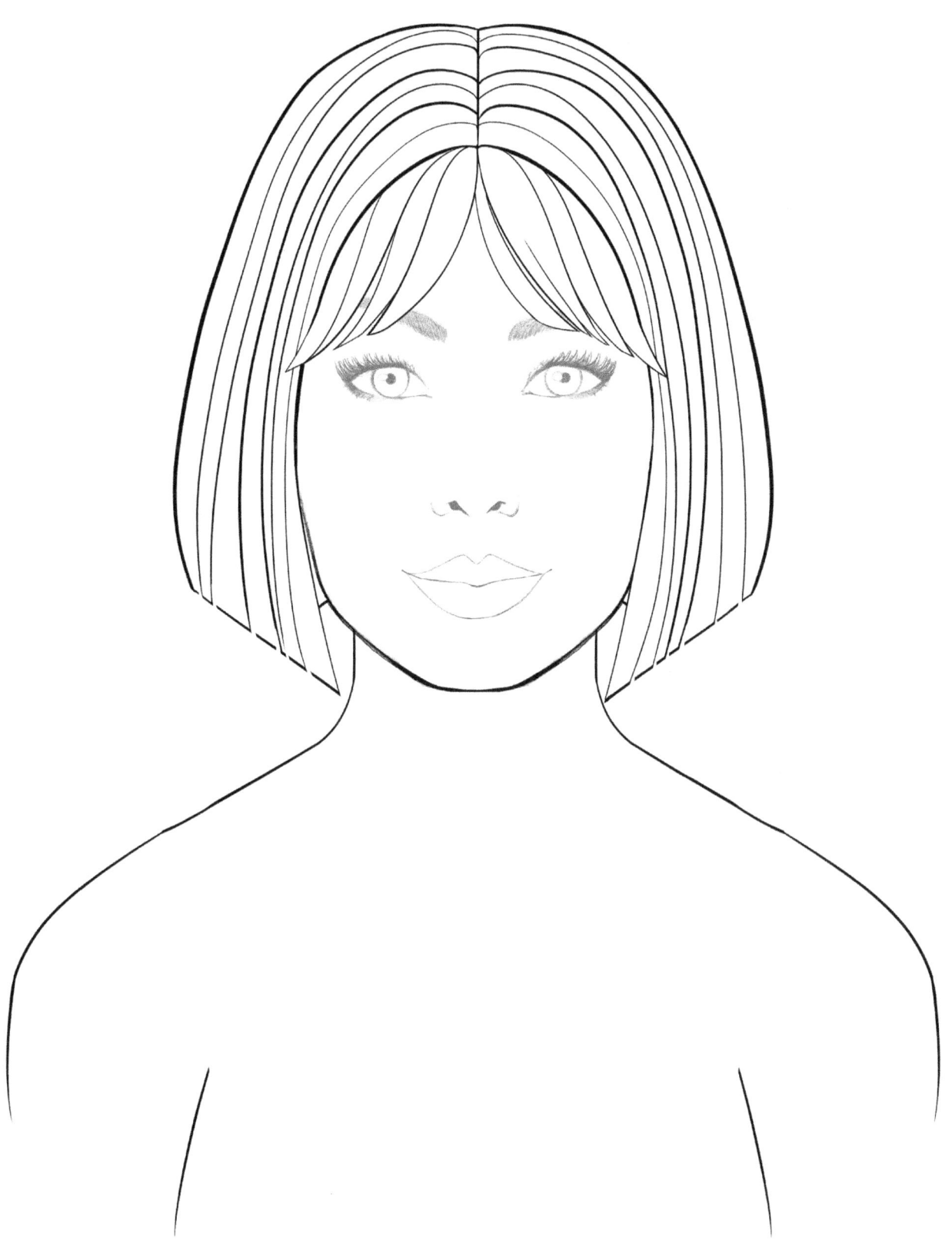

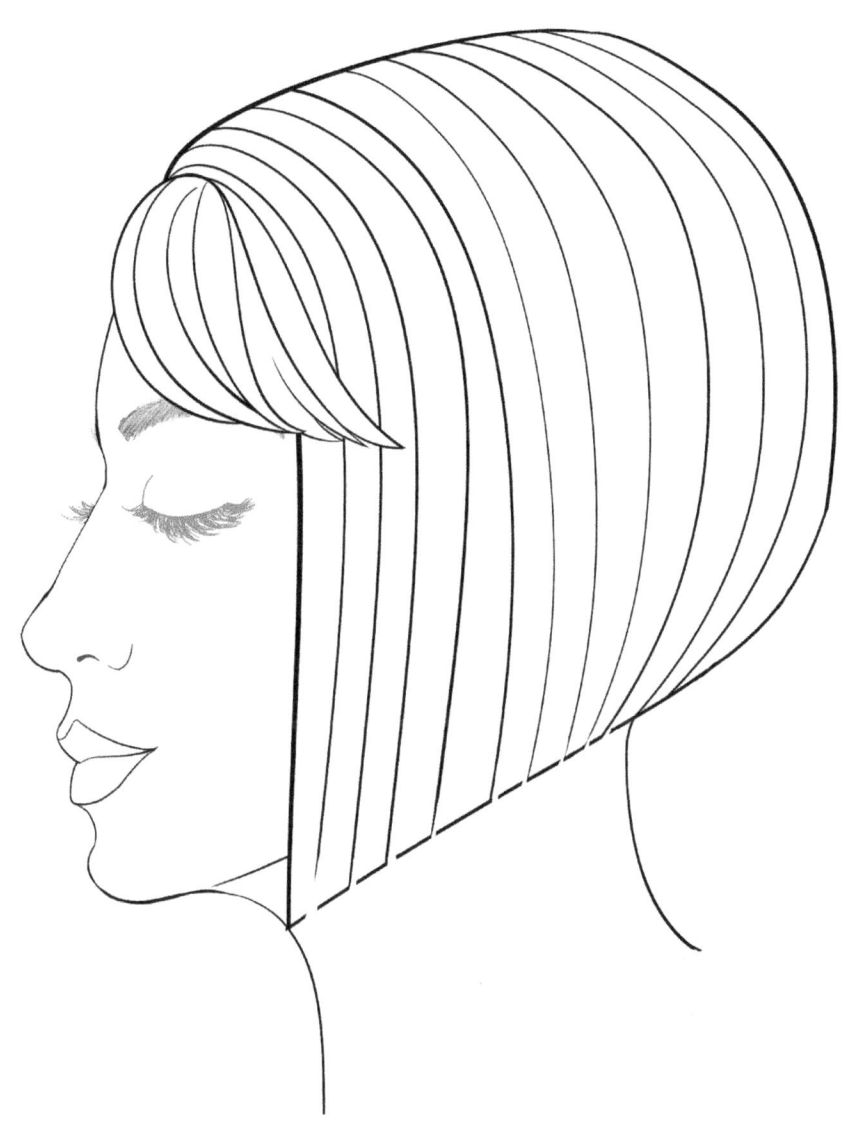

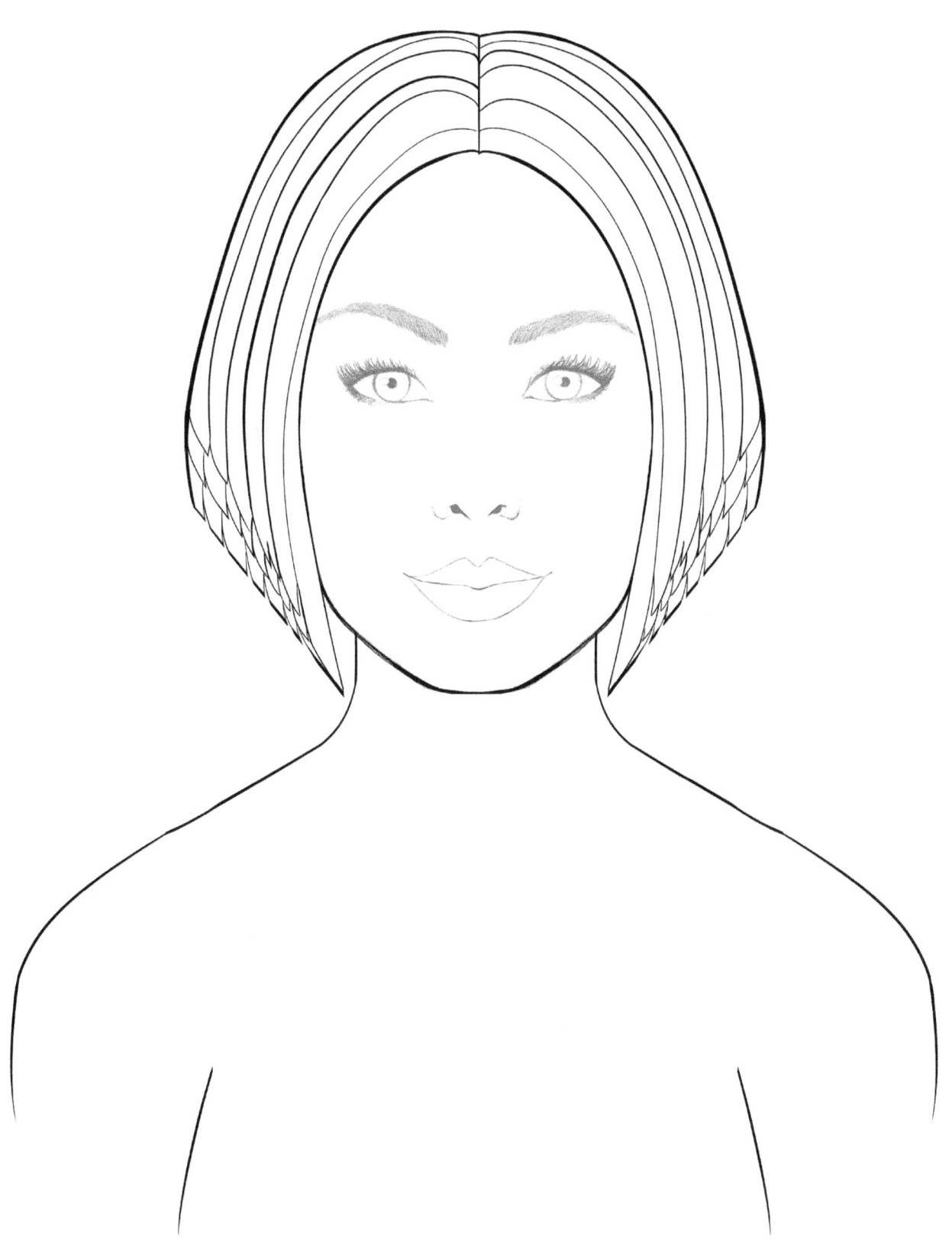

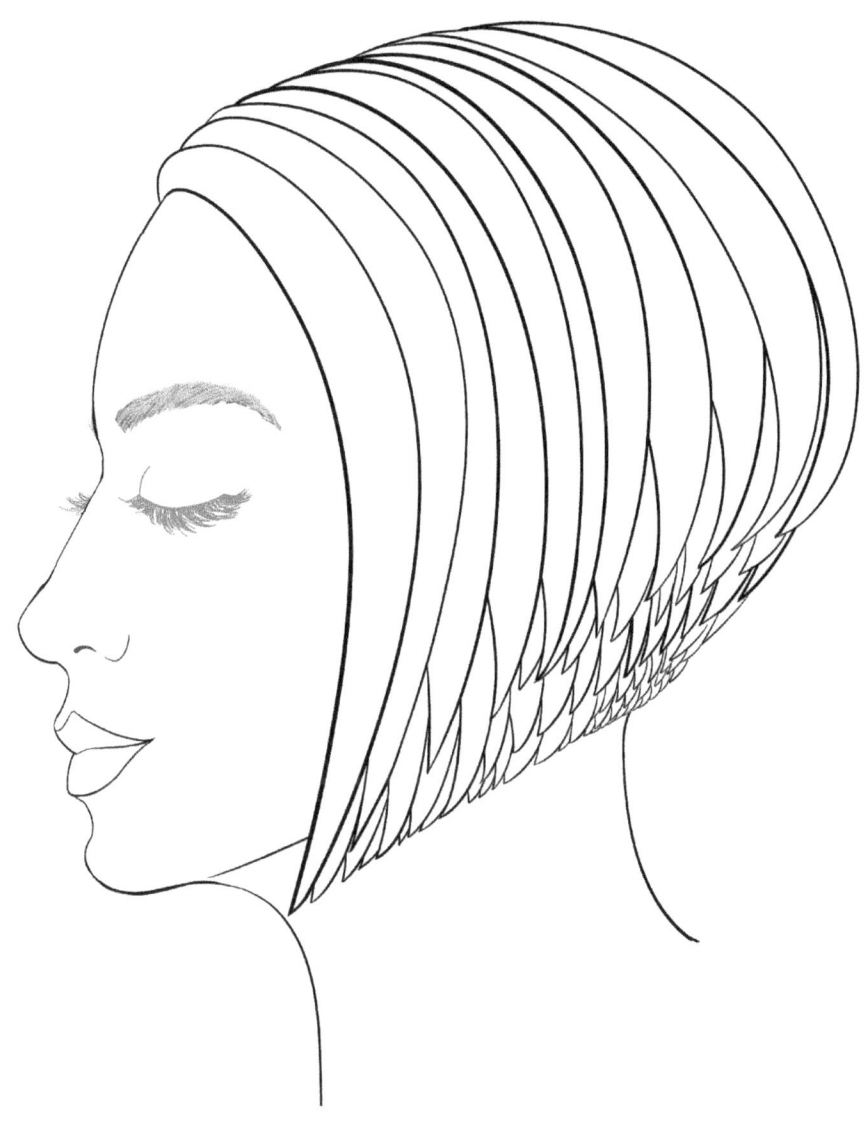

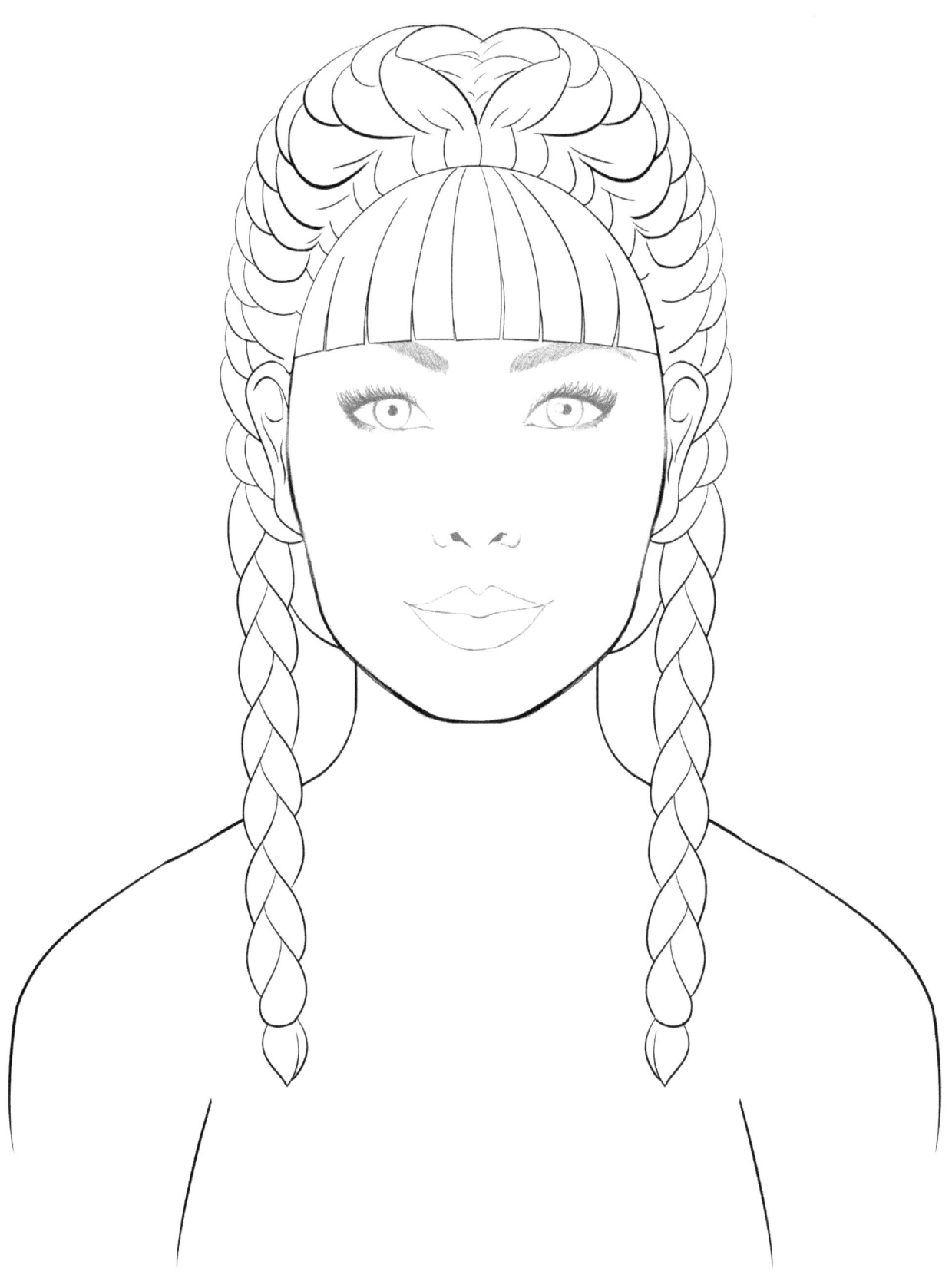

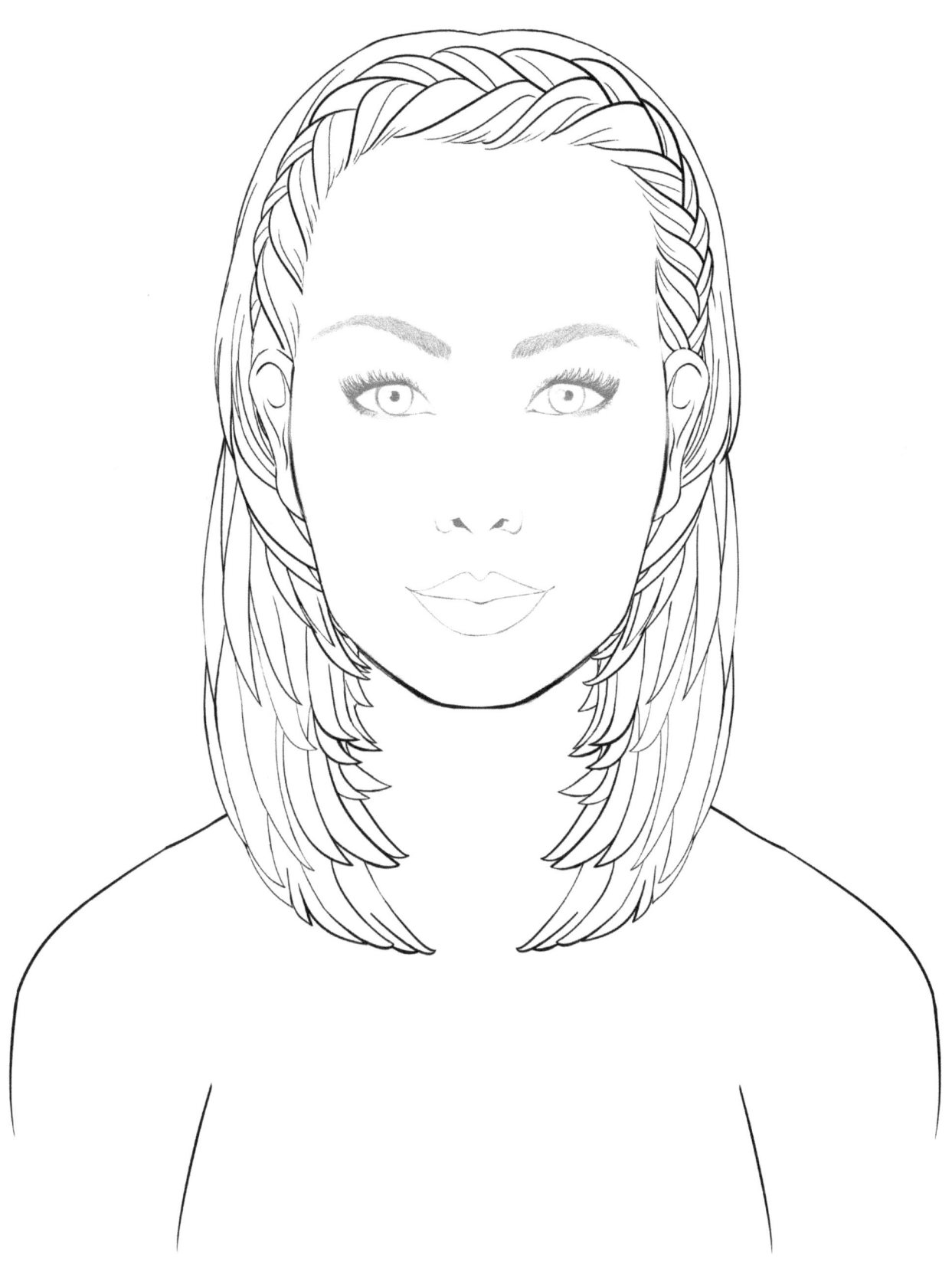

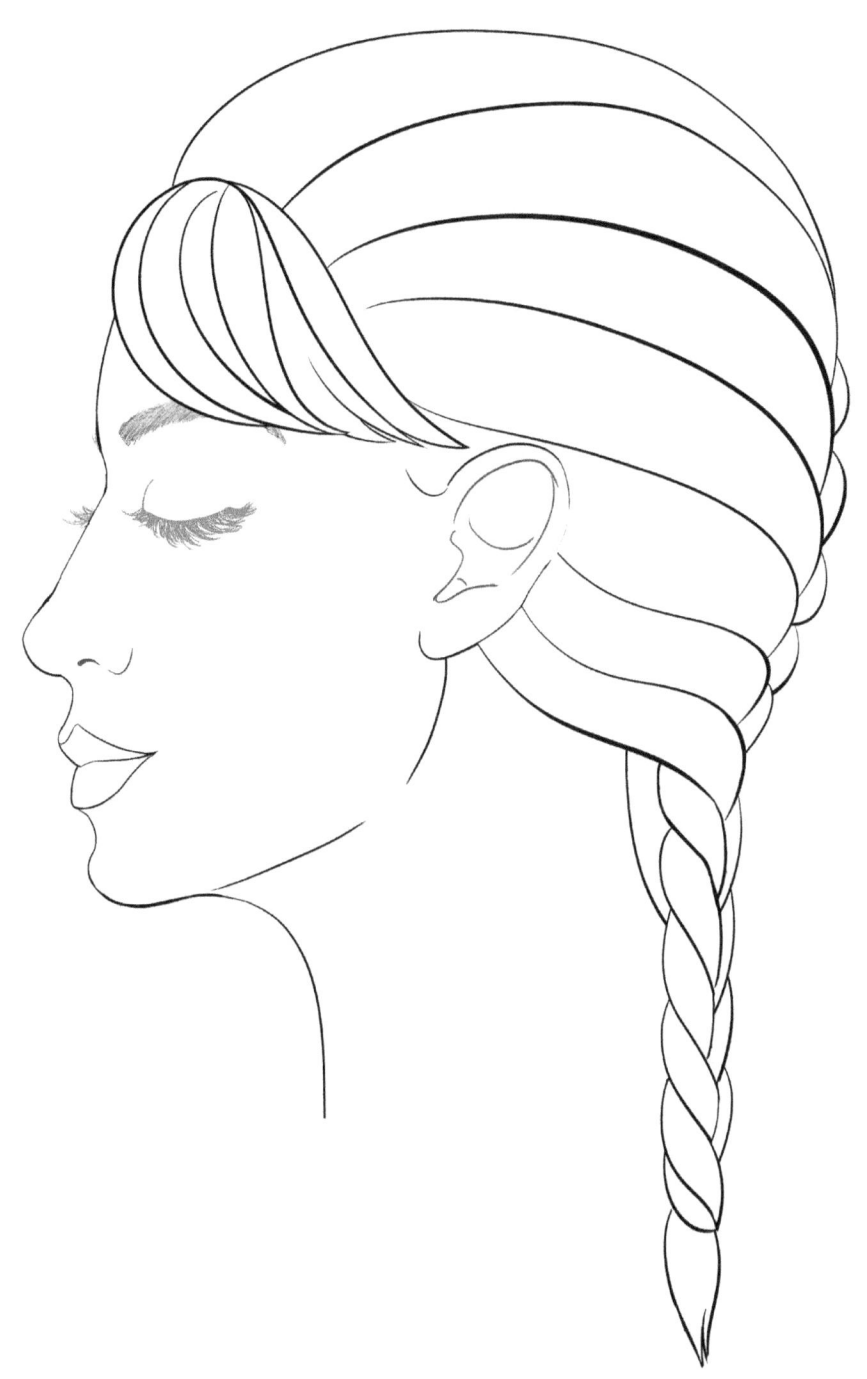

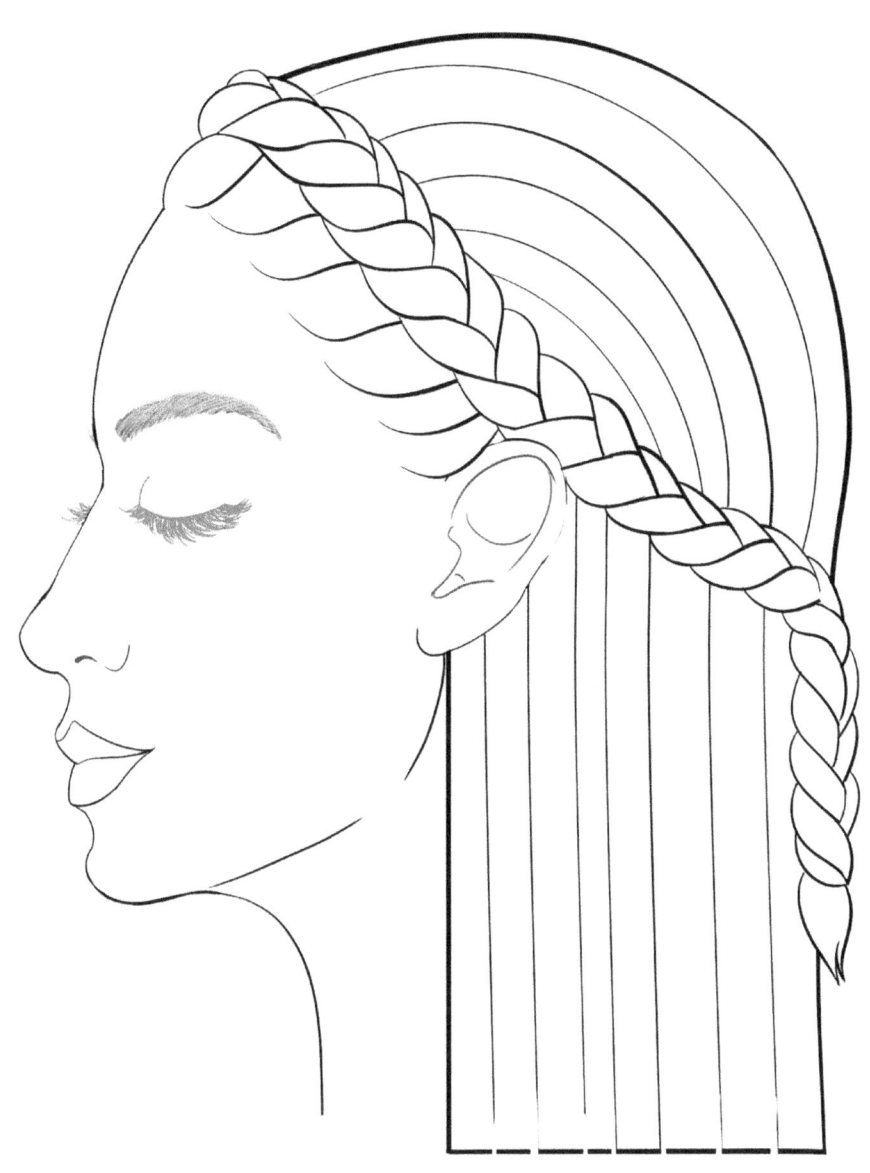

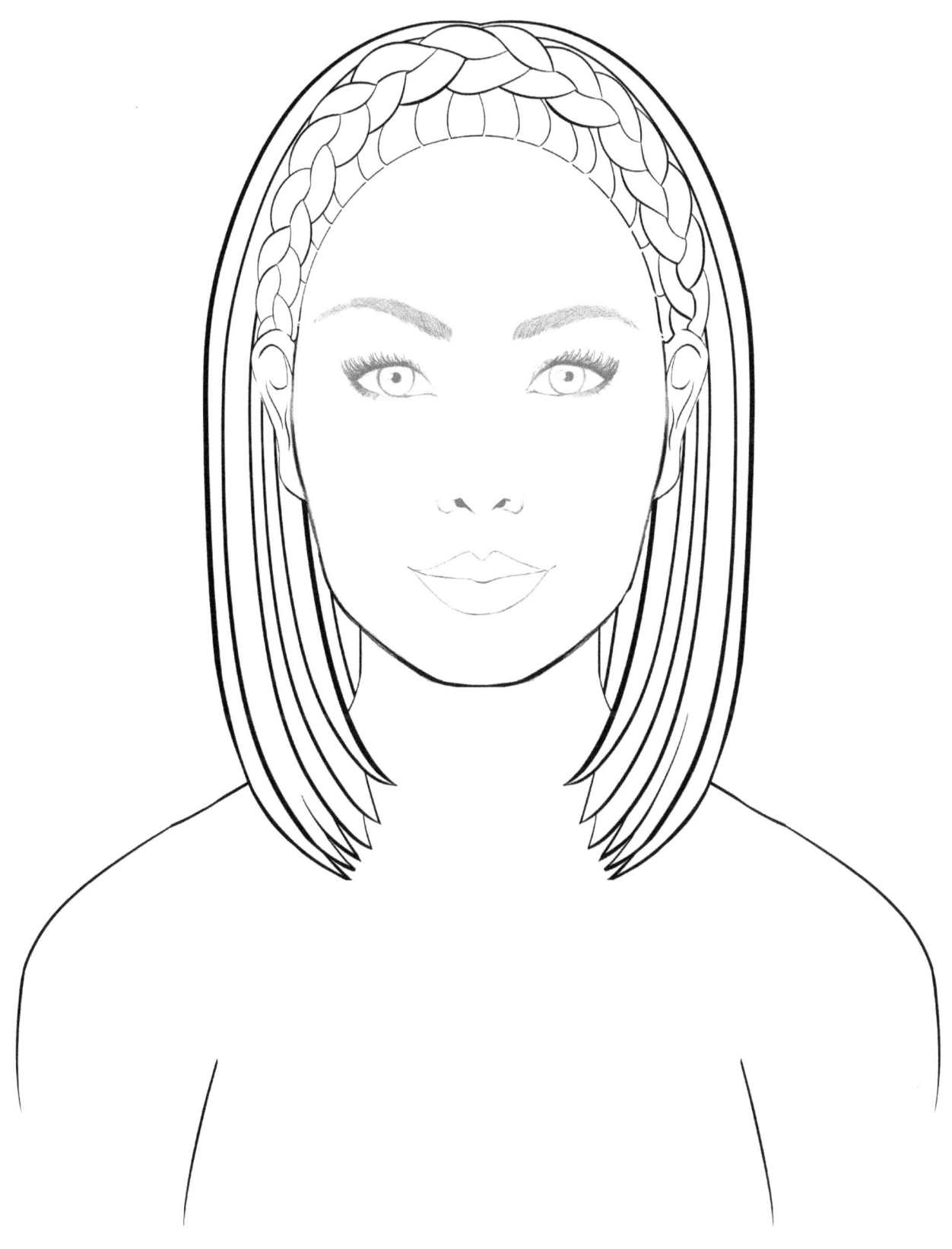

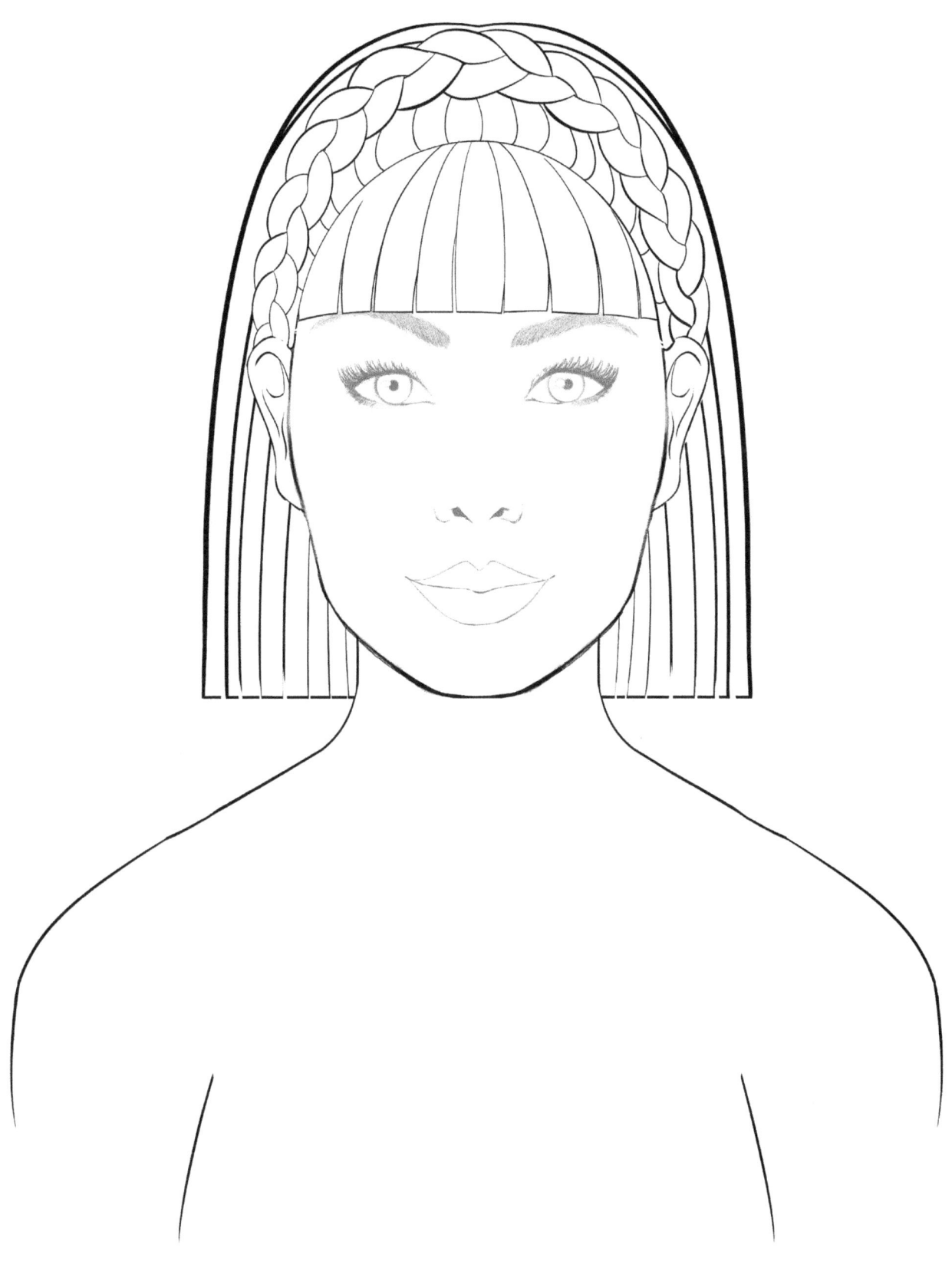

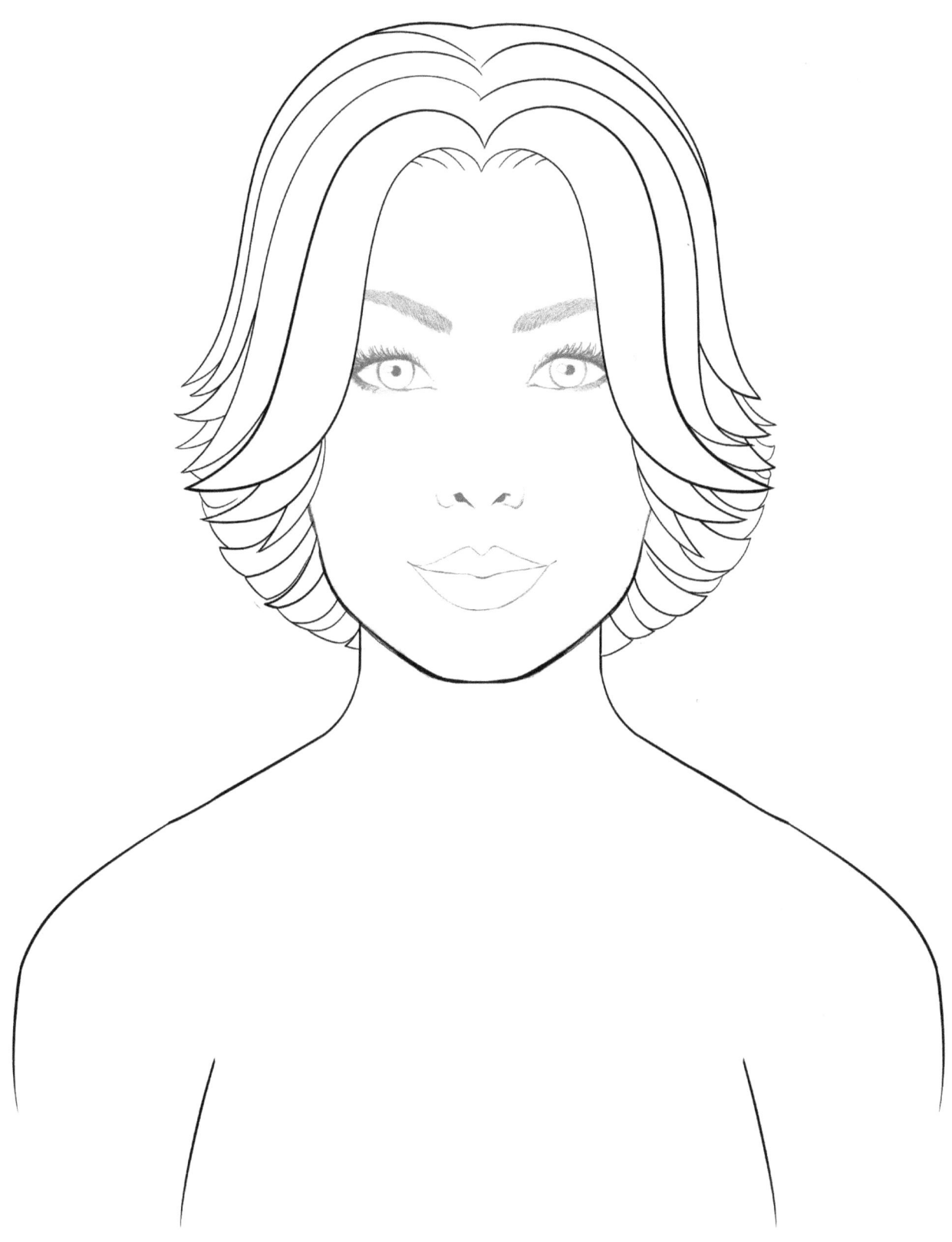

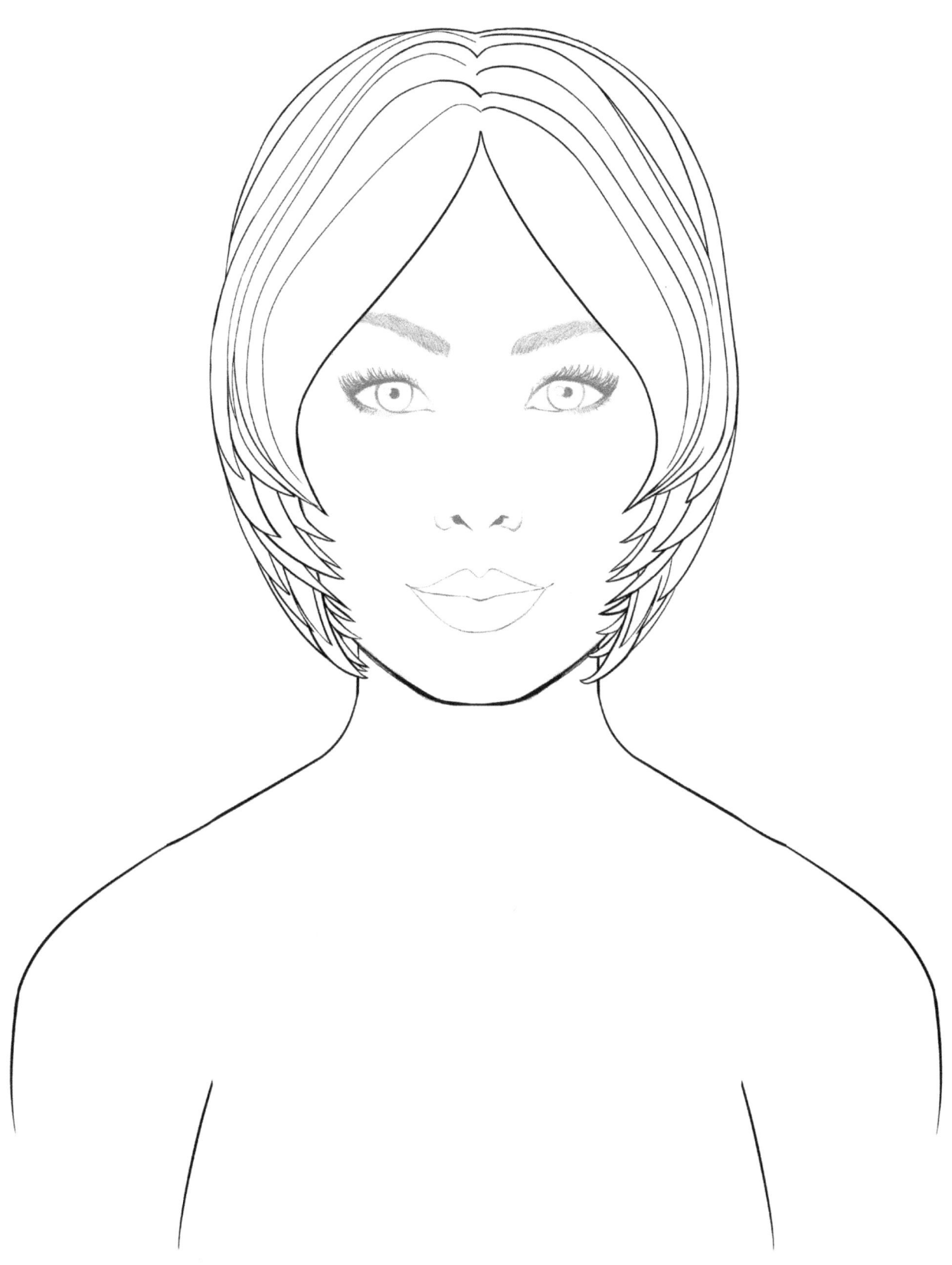

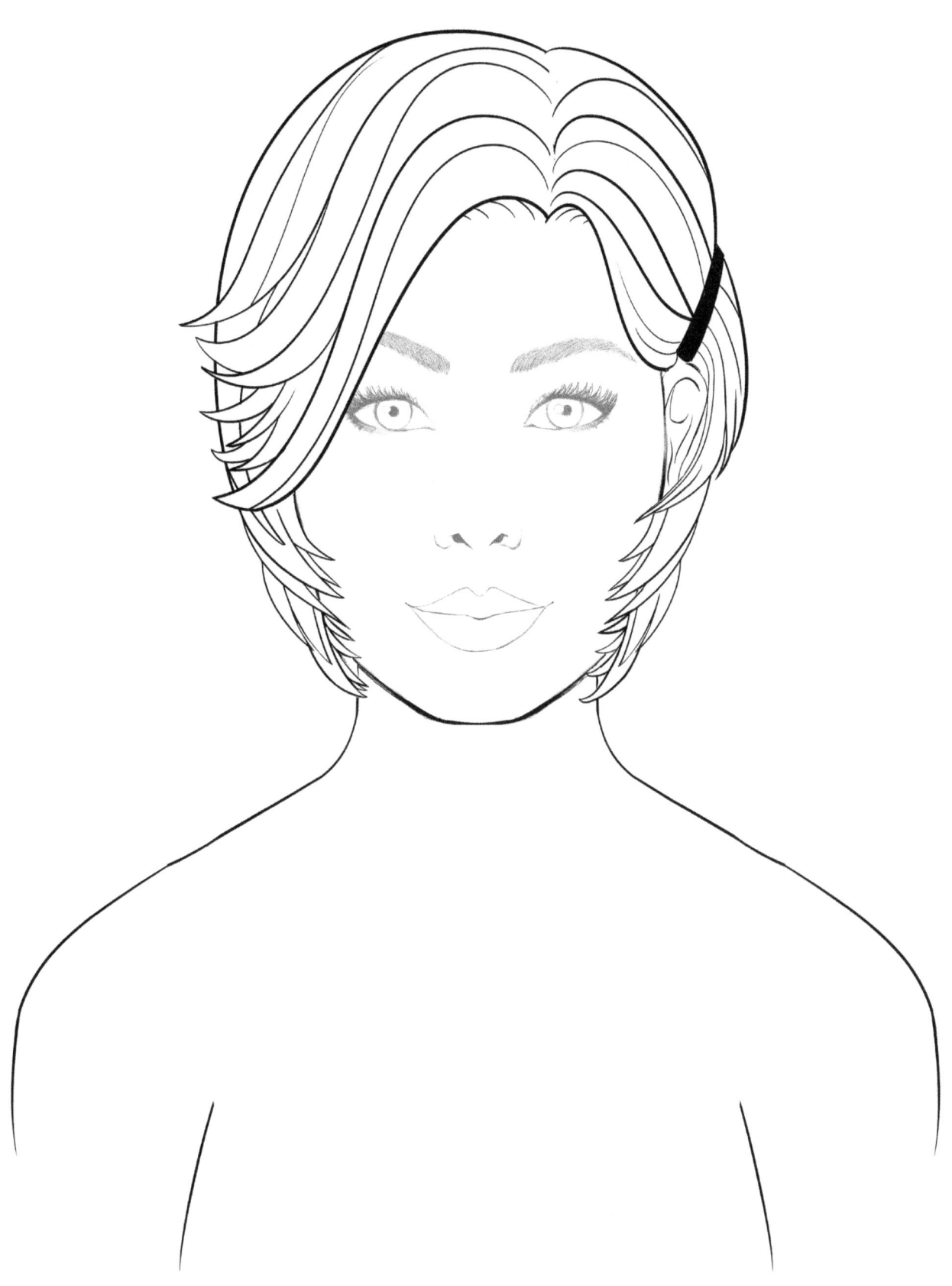

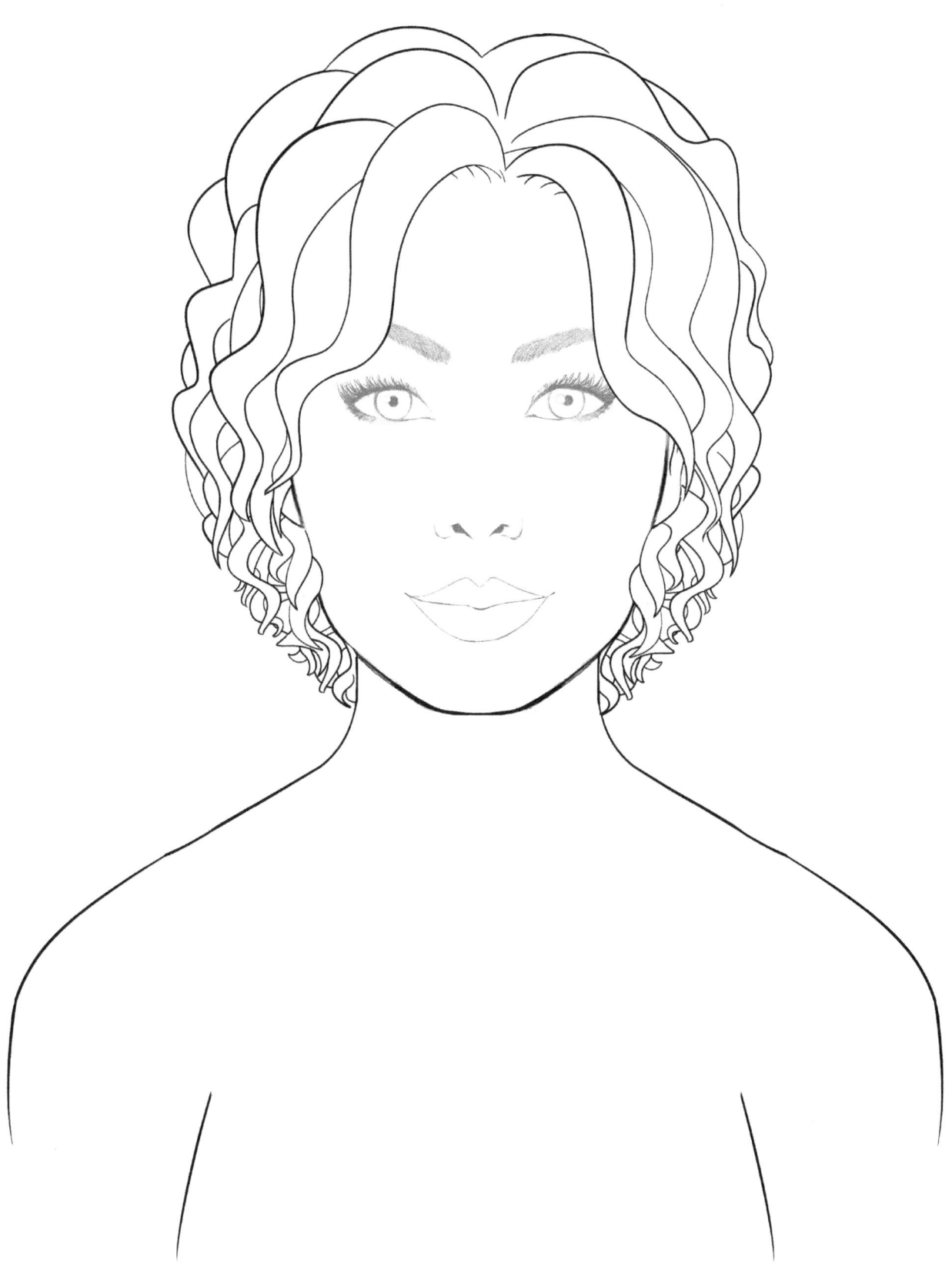

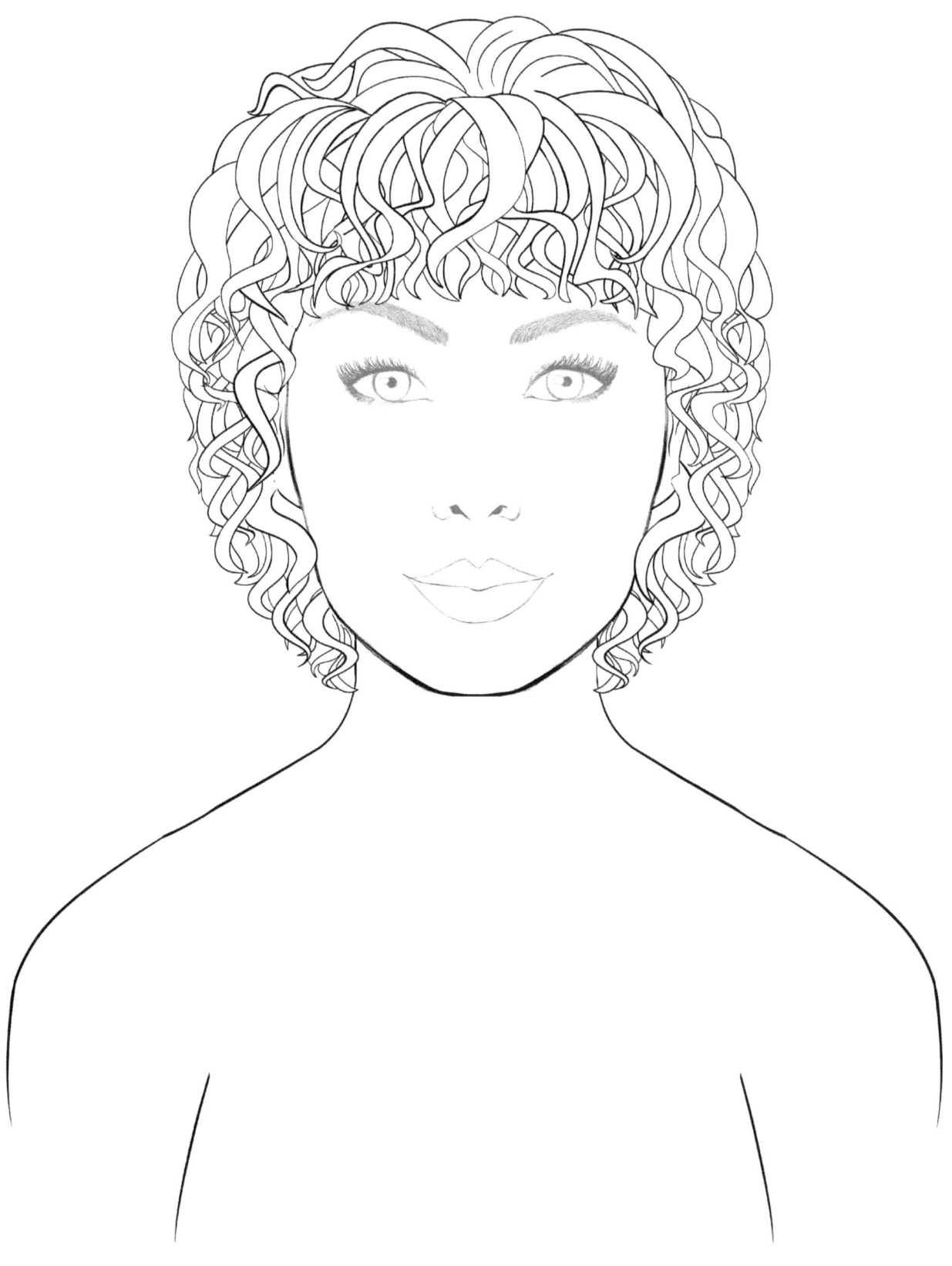

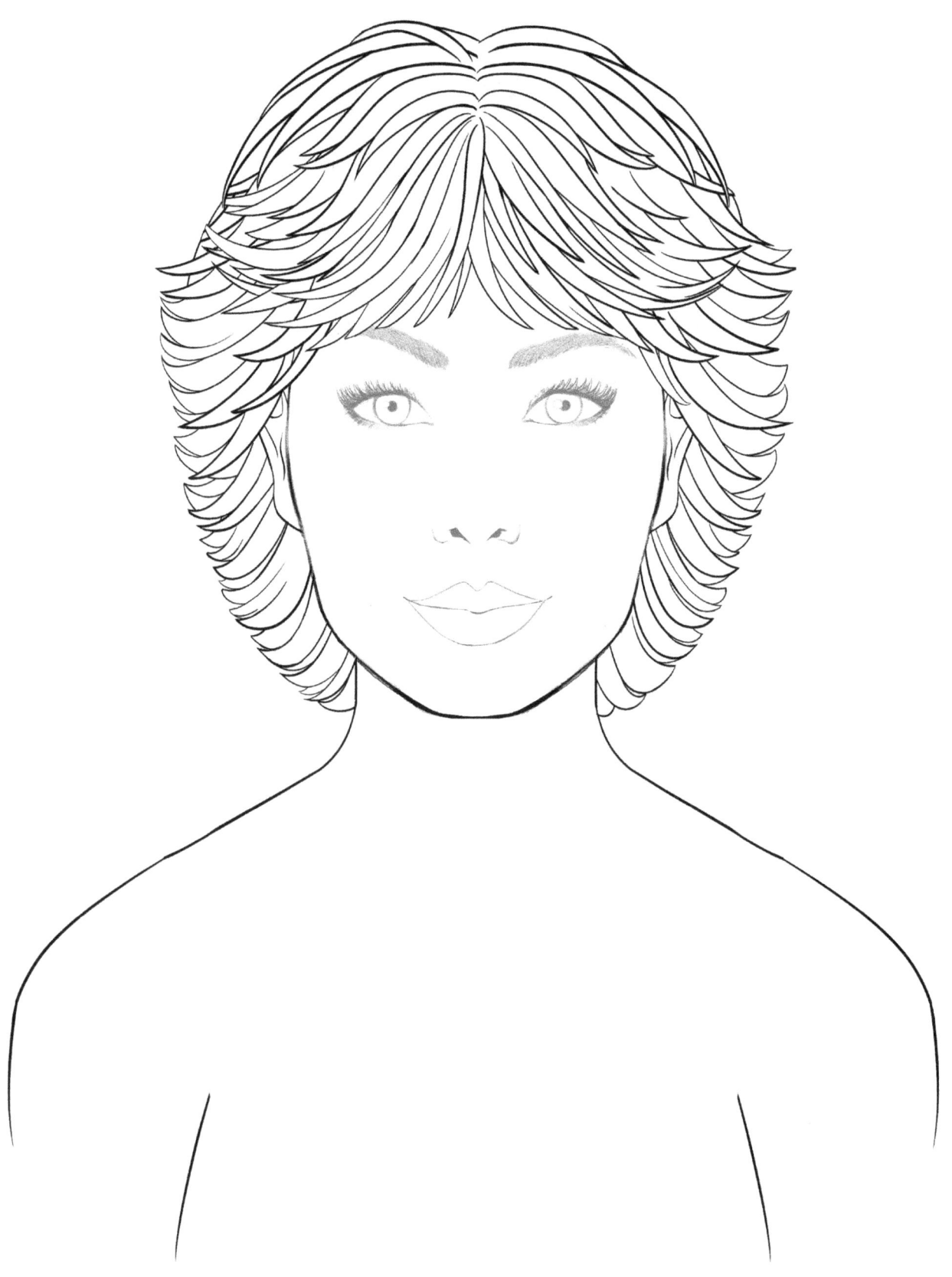

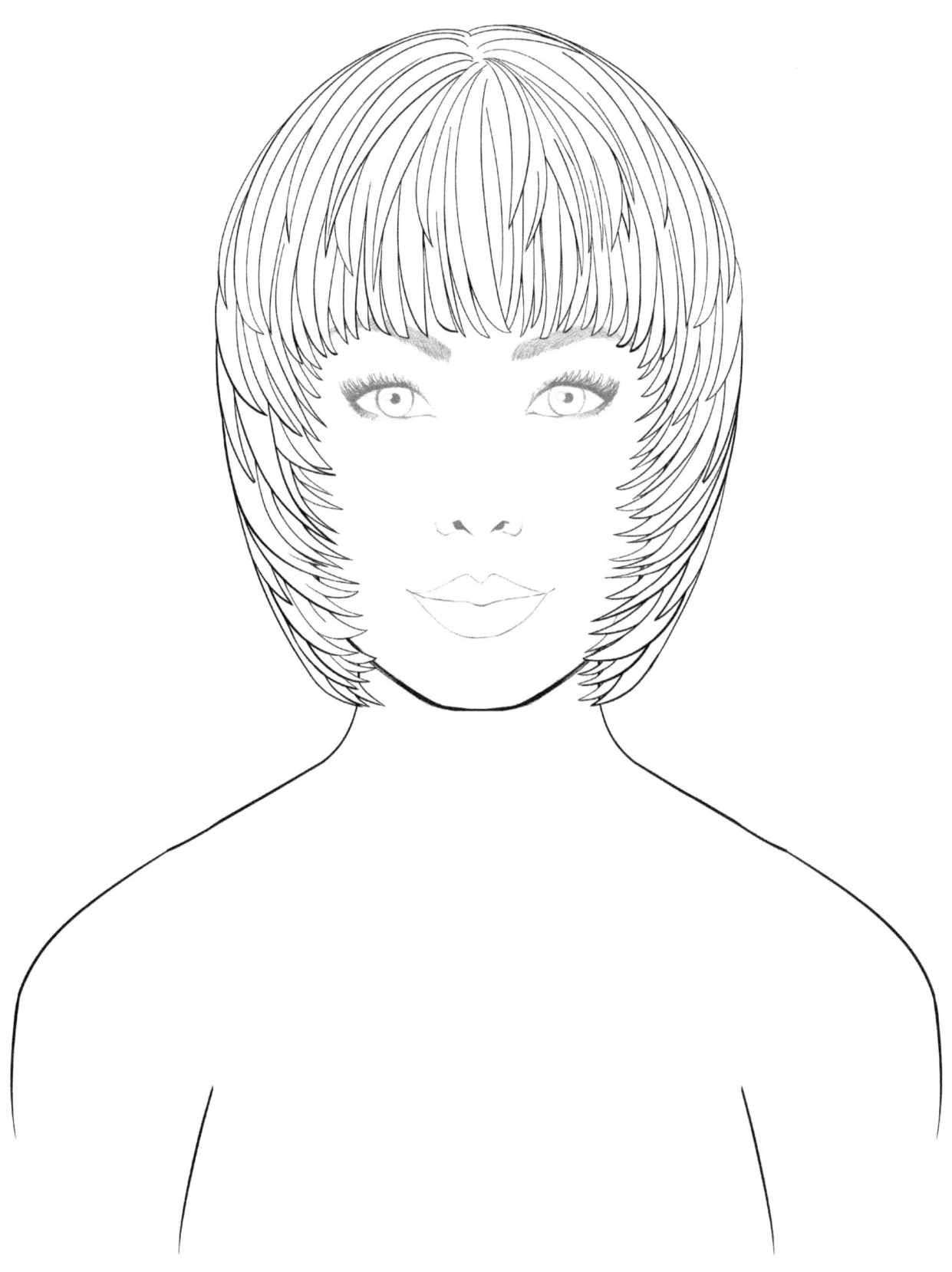

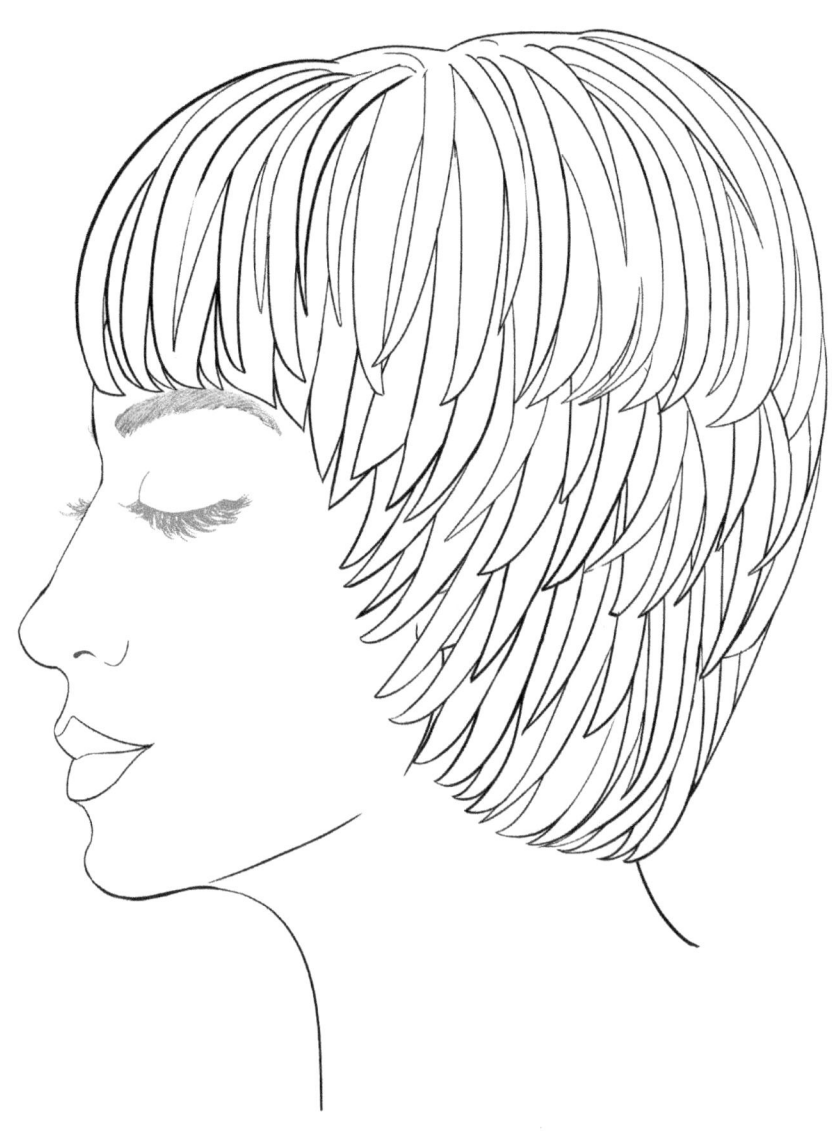

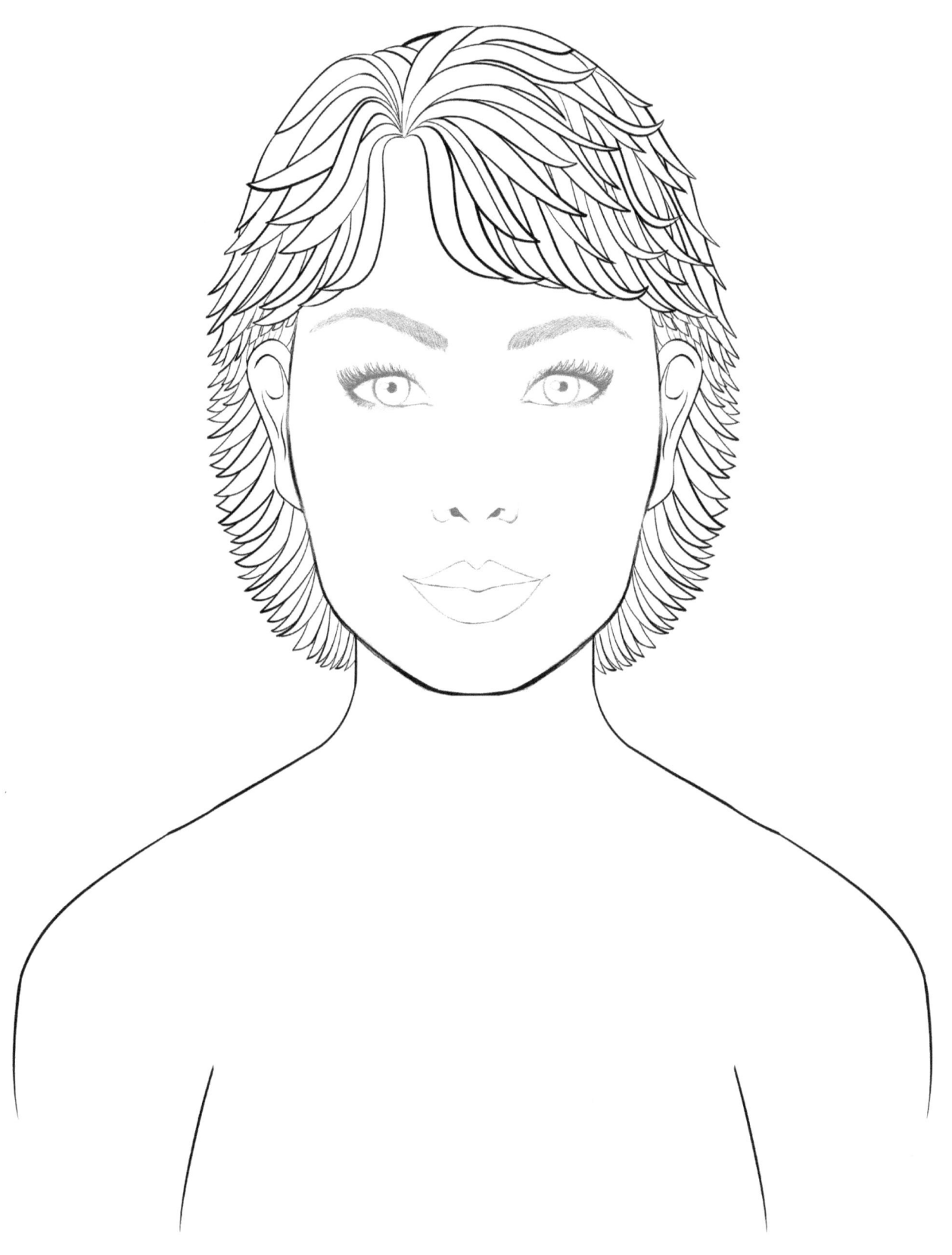

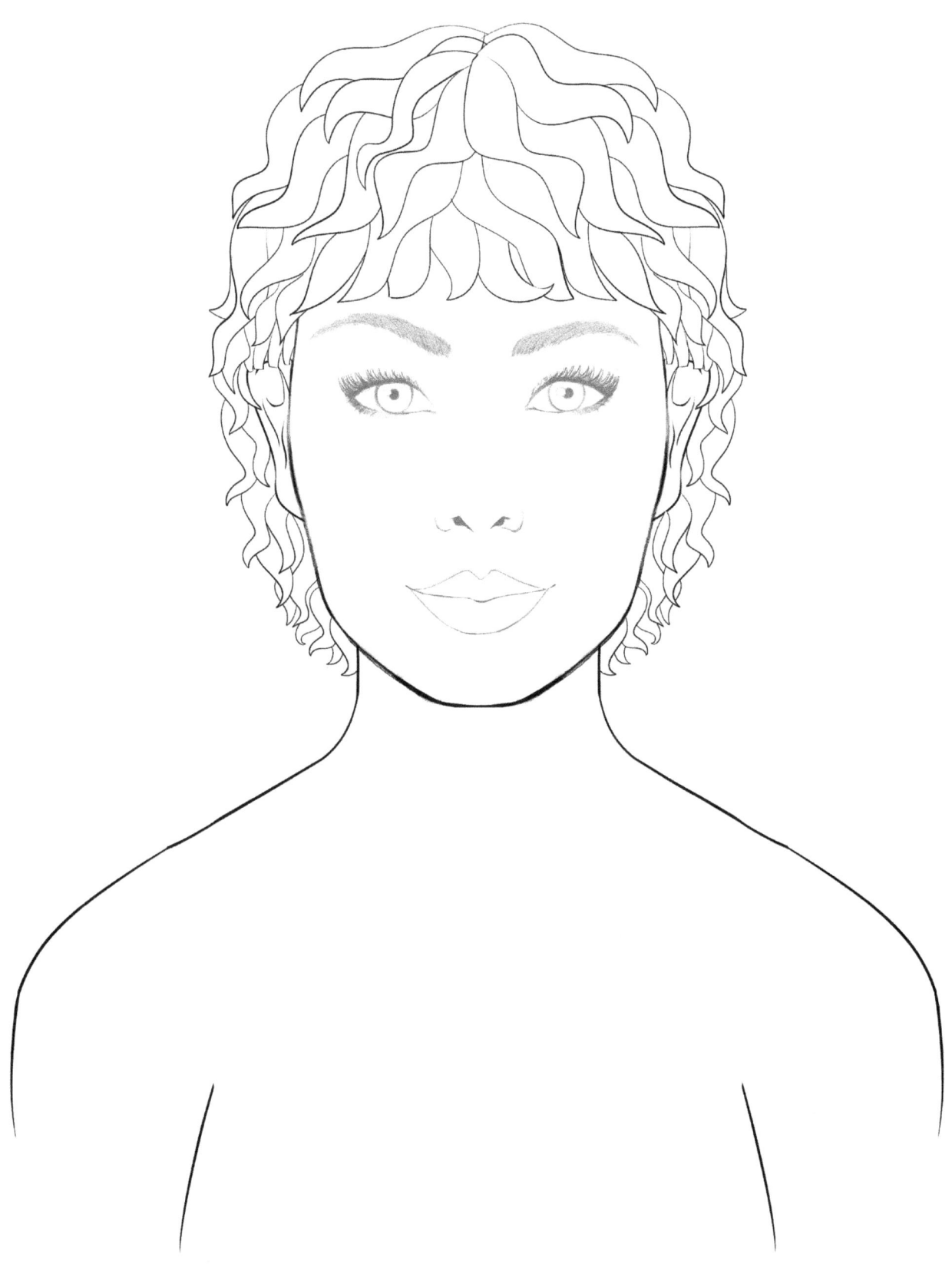

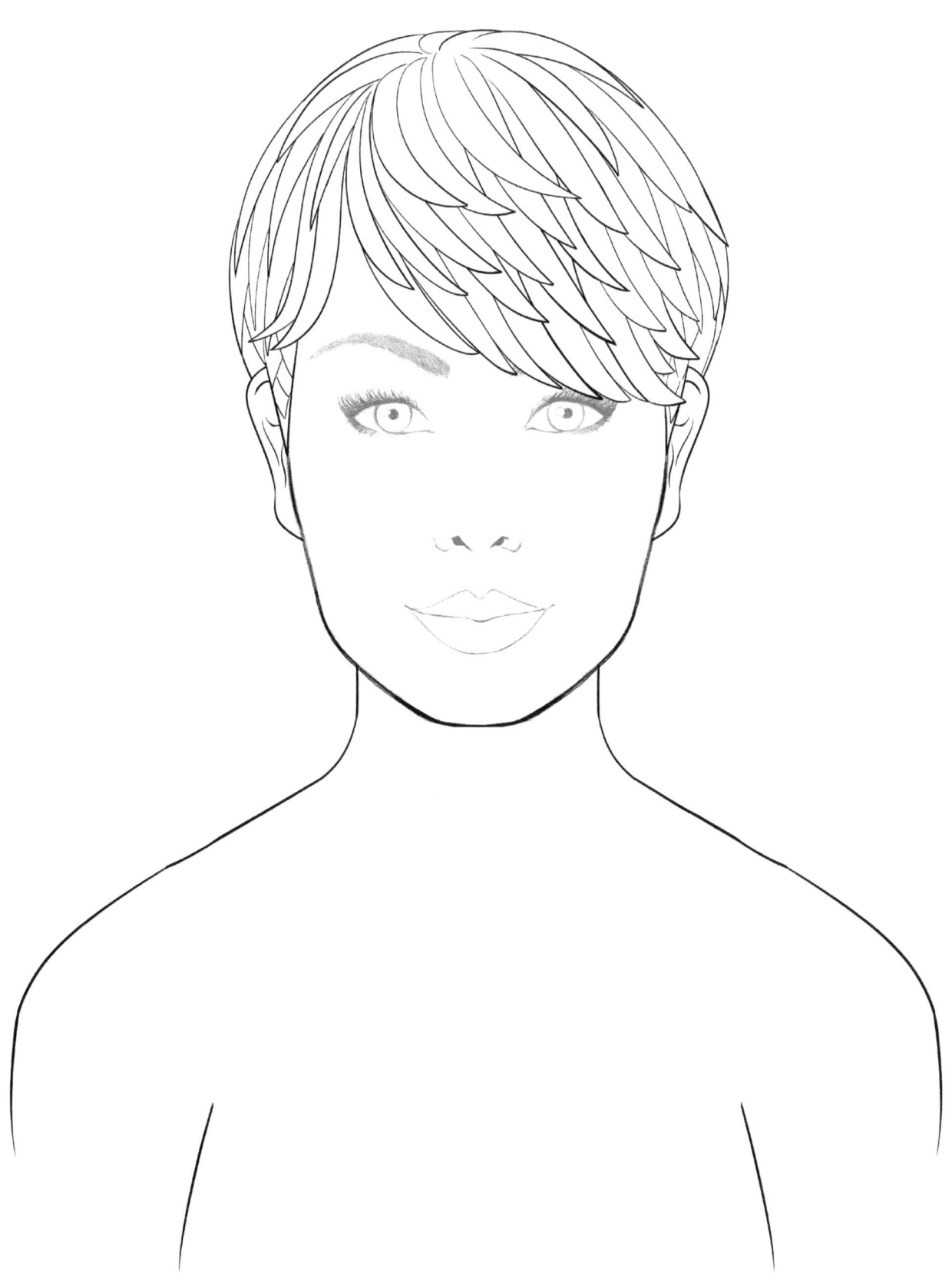

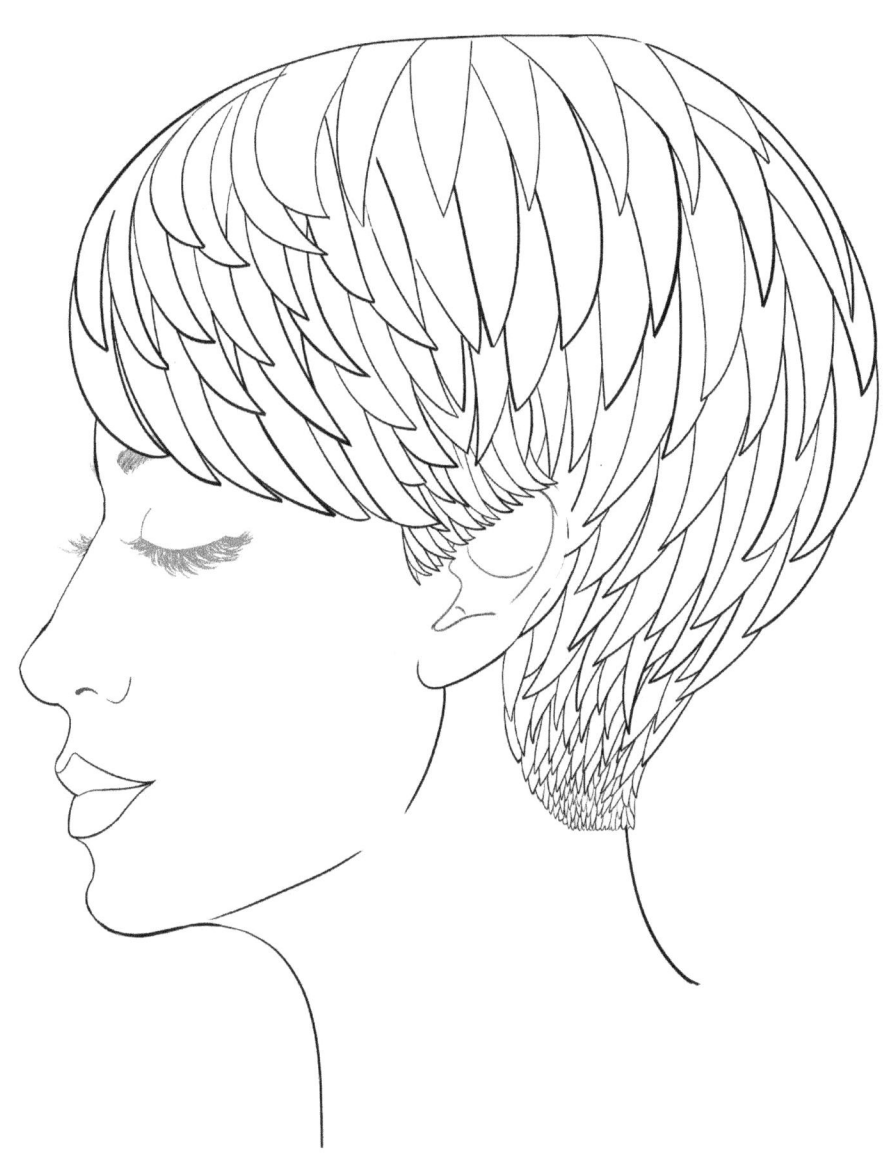

www.ingramcontent.com/pod-product-compliance
Lightning Source LLC
LaVergne TN
LVHW061937070526
838199LV00060B/3851

9798985039733